2025 EDITION

THE COMPLETE HOME APOTHECARY BOOK

401 EASY, STEP-BY-STEP
Herbal Remedies and Potent Blends to Relieve Pain, Boost Immunity, Improve Sleep, and Restore Balance Naturally

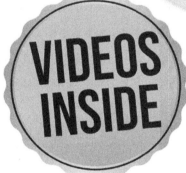

AVA GREEN

THE COMPLETE HOME APOTHECARY BOOK

Copyright © 2025 by Magnolia Publishing

All rights reserved.

No part of this publication may be reproduced, distributed, or transmitted in any form or by any means, including photocopying, recording, or other electronic or mechanical methods, without prior written permission from the publisher, except in the case of brief quotations used in reviews or for non-commercial purposes permitted by copyright law. This book is for informational purposes only. The author and publisher disclaim liability for any adverse effects resulting from the use or misuse of the information contained herein.

Disclaimer

The information in this book is based on the author's research, personal experience, and knowledge. It is not intended as a substitute for professional medical advice, diagnosis, or treatment. Always consult a licensed healthcare provider before using any herbal remedies, especially if you are pregnant, nursing, taking medication, or have preexisting conditions. While the author and publisher have made every effort to ensure the accuracy of the information, they are not responsible for errors, omissions, or outcomes related to the use of this book. Individual results may vary, and any use of the information is at your own risk.

FDA Disclaimer:

The statements in this book have not been evaluated by the Food and Drug Administration. The recipes and remedies provided are not intended to diagnose, treat, cure, or prevent any disease.

TABLE OF CONTENTS

PART 1: A STORY OF HEALING AND HOPE 1
Embracing Nature's Remedies 1
How Herbal Medicine Began 3
The Modern Age of Medicine 7

PART 2: THE HERBALIST'S GUIDE 10
Sourcing Ethically and Growing Effectively 10
The Importance of Correct Dosage 16
Best Forms for Herbal Effectiveness 19
The Herbal Initiation: 10 Sacred Starter Herbs for Beginners 26
Simple Yet Powerful Beginnings 37

PART 3: EXPANDING YOUR HERBAL KNOWLEDGE: ADDRESSING SPECIFIC AILMENTS 38
Herbs for Digestive Issues 39
Herbs for Respiratory Conditions 60
Herbs for Skin Conditions 82
Herbs for Stress and Anxiety 103
Herbs for Pain Management 125
Herbs for Immune Support 146
Herbs for Cardiovascular Health 167
Herbs for Detoxification 189
Herbs for Hormonal Imbalances 211
Herbs for Mental Clarity 232

HERBAL GLOSSARY 255

PART 1
A STORY OF HEALING AND HOPE

EMBRACING NATURE'S REMEDIES

People often ask how I came to know so much about herbs. The truth is, it's been a lifelong journey rooted in curiosity, experience, and a deep connection to nature. As a child, I spent every free moment outdoors, exploring the plants around me. My grandmother was my first teacher, introducing me to the wildflowers she knew so well. She would take me out into the fields and show me how to recognize their shapes, smells, and uses. Her wisdom came from years of experience, and she shared it with me in a way that felt both gentle and profound. I'd kneel by her side as she sorted herbs from her garden, learning which plants were for healing, which were for cooking, and which belonged in the compost.

Her garden was like a living pharmacy, and the time I spent there felt magical. I wasn't just learning about plants—I was learning how to observe, to respect, and to connect with nature. As the years passed, my fascination with plants only deepened. I began to see them not just as part of the landscape but as living allies with unique abilities to heal, nourish, and transform. My grandmother's lessons became the foundation for my own explorations. I would pore over field guides during the winter, memorizing the characteristics of plants I hoped to find when spring arrived. By the time the snow melted, I'd have a mental list of plants I wanted to seek out, armed with the excitement of discovering them in the wild.

By the time I was in middle school, I was making my own herbal remedies. At first, it was simple things: teas for colds, salves for cuts and scrapes. But as my confidence grew, I began sharing these remedies with others. Friends and family started asking for advice or for something to help with an ache, a cough, or a sleepless night. I realized then that the knowledge my grandmother had passed down wasn't just a skill—it was a gift—and one I could share with others to make a difference in their lives.

Herbalism became more than a hobby; it was a way of life. It wasn't just about the remedies—it was about the connection to the earth, the understanding that everything we need to heal and thrive is provided by nature if we take the time to learn and respect it. My grandmother used to say, "The plants will always tell you what they're for if you're willing to listen." That phrase stayed with me, guiding my work and my approach to herbalism. And this is how this manual came to be.

For those just starting their herbal journey, the world of plants may seem overwhelming. But most herbalists rely on a small number of plants for daily use. Begin with one or two herbs, get to know them deeply, and experiment with how to use them. Whether you're brewing tea, making salves, or simply sitting with a plant, every step strengthens your connection to herbalism.

This book is designed to guide you on that journey. Inside, you'll find profiles of potent medicinal plants, practical advice, and natural therapies that support your body, mind, and spirit. My goal is to share the knowledge that I've gained over the years, blending traditional wisdom, modern science behind the chemicals that make these plants effective, and my own experiences to inspire your own exploration into the healing power of herbs. Whether you're new to herbalism or have years of experience, there's always more to learn—and I'm thrilled to take this journey with you.

HOW HERBAL MEDICINE BEGAN

Herbal wisdom traces back to humanity's earliest days as hunters and gatherers living off the land. Over time, people discovered that certain plants held special properties. These herbs could heal wounds, cure diseases, and even, they believed, protect against evil spirits. Guided by shamans, early societies viewed herbs as sacred gifts from the gods, using them in rituals, ceremonies, and as powerful remedies when combined with animal parts and minerals.

In ancient Egypt, around 2667–2648 BCE, a man named Imhotep emerged as the earliest known physician, laying the foundations of Egyptian medicine. The Egyptians revered herbs like thyme, fennel, aloe, and myrrh—not only for their medicinal qualities but also for their spiritual significance. Garlic and onions, prized for their ability to enhance strength and endurance, were so valued that they were placed in the tombs of pharaohs to aid them in the afterlife.

Meanwhile, in Mesopotamia, medical practices advanced with the creation of one of the first diagnostic handbooks. This early text allowed doctors to systematically diagnose illnesses and prescribe treatments, marking a pivotal step in the organization of medicine.

Ayurveda: The Mother of All Medicine

As centuries passed, civilizations around the world developed their own systems of medicine, each deeply rooted in the healing power of herbs. In India, Ayurveda emerged over 5,000 years ago, often called the "mother of all medicine." Ayurveda emphasized the balance of physical, mental, and spiritual well-being, achieved through specific herbs, diets, and lifestyle practices.

According to tradition, the mythical physician Dhanvantari, said to have learned Ayurveda from the god Brahma, served as the healer to the gods. Initially passed down orally, Ayurvedic teachings were later recorded in the Vedas, particularly the Atharvaveda. Composed around the second millennium BCE, these texts blended herbal remedies with spiritual practices, addressing ailments such as fever, cough, tumors, and skin diseases with a wide array of plants.

Golden Era of Indian Medicine

Between 1000 BCE and 800 BCE, the golden era of Indian medicine produced two foundational texts: the *Charaka Samhita*, attributed to the physician Charaka, and the *Sushruta Samhita*, authored by the surgeon Suśruta. These works detailed the elements of earth, water, fire, air, and ether, alongside the bodily humors of vata, pitta, and kapha. Together, they laid the groundwork for subsequent Indian medical knowledge, offering profound insights into the interconnectedness of body, mind, and nature.

Traditional Chinese Medicine: Balancing Yin and Yang

Meanwhile, in China, another ancient system of medicine took shape: traditional Chinese medicine (TCM). With roots stretching back over 5,000 years, its foundational text, the *Huangdi Neijing* (Yellow Emperor's Inner Classic), was compiled around the third century BCE.

This text introduced principles still central to TCM today, emphasizing the balance of yin (passive energy) and yang (active energy) as essential to health. Imbalance between these forces, it taught, led to illness. Traditional Chinese pharmacies were repositories of nature's remedies. Filled with rows of jars and drawers containing dried plants, minerals, and animal parts, they were a reflection of TCM's holistic approach.

The *Bencao Gangmu* (Compendium of Materia Medica), written in 1578 by Li Shizhen, cataloged nearly 1,900 medicines and 11,000 prescriptions, underscoring the vast scope of Chinese herbal knowledge. Central to TCM is the concept of qi (life force), which flows through meridians—channels connecting the body's organs and systems. To restore balance and promote health, TCM practitioners use a variety of techniques, including:

- Acupuncture: Thin needles inserted into specific points on the body to stimulate qi flow.
- Moxibustion: Burning herbs near the skin to encourage healing.
- Herbal Formulas: Carefully crafted combinations of herbs tailored to harmonize the body's energy.

In TCM, every part of a plant is classified for its medicinal properties, and even food is considered for its healing energies. For example, certain foods are believed to target specific organs, reinforcing TCM's holistic view that diet and medicine are deeply intertwined.

The Greeks and the Birth of Western Medicine

Then, around 700 BCE, the Greeks began to explore the healing arts in earnest. They told stories of the gods Apollo and Asclepius, who were believed to have passed down the knowledge of herbs and medicine. According to legend, Apollo rescued the unborn Asclepius from his mother's funeral pyre and placed him in the care of the wise centaur Chiron. Chiron was well known for his expertise in herbal medicine, and he taught Asclepius everything he knew.

Asclepius became so skilled in the art of healing that he was said to have used the blood of the gorgon to bring the dead back to life. This power made Zeus jealous. He struck Asclepius down with a thunderbolt. But Asclepius was not forgotten; he became the Greek god of healing. His knowledge of herbs was passed down through the generations.

One of the most famous students of this tradition was Hippocrates, who lived around 460–370 BCE. Hippocrates is often called the "father of modern medicine" because he rejected the magical remedies of the past. Instead, he focused on careful observation and the use of "herbal simples"—single herbs used as medicine. He compiled lengthy inventory of medicinal herbs, many of which are still used today. Hippocrates believed that herbs could cure most ailments. His teachings laid the groundwork for the development of a true science of medicine.

The Spread of Herbal Knowledge

As the Greek and Roman empires expanded, so did their knowledge of herbs. The Romans, in particular, were known for their use of herbs like rosemary and bay leaf, which they used not only in cooking but also in rituals and ceremonies. Roman soldiers carried these herbs with them as they conquered new lands. In this way, they spread their use throughout Europe.

In the centuries that followed, much of the knowledge of herbs was preserved by monks in European monasteries. During the Dark Ages (500–1000 CE), these monks cultivated herb gardens and copied ancient texts. They ensured that the wisdom of the past would not be lost.

One of the most famous of these texts is *Bald's Leechbook*, a ninth-century collection of remedies that includes both physical cures and incantations to drive away evil spirits.

As trade routes expanded, so did the exchange of herbal knowledge. The Silk Road, which connected Europe to Asia, brought new herbs and spices to the West. Italian adventurers like Marco Polo brought back tales of exotic plants from the East, and European merchants quickly realized the value of these herbs.

The Renaissance and the Printing Revolution

The 15th century marked a turning point in the history of herbal medicine with the invention of the printing press. This revolutionary technology enabled the mass production of books, including works on herbal remedies. For the first time, ordinary people could access knowledge that had previously been restricted to scholars and the elite.

One of the most influential figures to emerge during this period was Nicholas Culpeper, an English herbalist and botanist of the 17th century. Culpeper made medical knowledge accessible to the public by translating the *London Pharmacopeia* from Latin into English. His work empowered people to take control of their health, providing herbal formulas that could be created using plants grown in their own gardens.

Culpeper's Herbal, published in 1653, became a household staple and a symbol of self-reliance. Its popularity extended across the Atlantic, where early Puritan settlers brought it to the American colonies, ensuring the survival of herbal traditions in the New World.

Herbal Medicine in the New World

When the colonists arrived in America, they brought with them the herbs, practices, and knowledge of the Old World. However, they also encountered an entirely new array of plants and ideas from Native Americans, who had their own rich and deeply rooted traditions of herbal medicine. This exchange of knowledge led to a unique system of herbal practice, blending centuries of wisdom from both sides of the Atlantic.

Herbs like thyme, lavender, and rosemary quickly became staples in colonial gardens, valued not only for their culinary uses but also for their medicinal properties. These versatile plants were essential in treating a variety of ailments, from digestive issues to infections, and played an integral role in the settlers' everyday lives. The merging of European and Native American herbal traditions created a vibrant and practical approach to healing, rooted in the natural resources of the New World.

THE MODERN AGE OF MEDICINE

In the early 19th century, a groundbreaking shift occurred in medicine. Scientists began using chemical analysis to isolate the active components of plants, leading to the creation of synthetic medicines. These laboratory-produced drugs could be mass-manufactured, offering consistent dosages and quicker results. As pharmaceuticals became more widespread, the use of herbal remedies gradually declined.

Yet, even today, plants remain foundational to modern medicine. Over a quarter of pharmaceutical drugs derive their active ingredients from plants, a testament to the enduring power and wisdom of nature.

However, in our embrace of modern medicine, we have lost some of our connection to the plants themselves. Herbalists like Jen Bredesen of the California School of Herbal Studies emphasize the value of using the whole plant rather than isolated chemicals. Herbs offer more than physical healing; they forge a bond between us and the earth, connecting us to our ancestors and reminding us of nature's profound role in our well-being. The two trains of thought of herbal and modern, conventional medicine vary significantly in their methods, philosophy, and understanding of health.

Herbal Medicine: A Holistic Perspective

Herbal medicine focuses on treating the whole person—not just the symptoms of disease but also the underlying causes, emotional well-being, and spiritual balance. It views the body as an interconnected system where every part influences the whole, and healing is achieved by restoring balance. Remedies are often tailored to the individual, considering their constitution, lifestyle, and emotional state.

Modern Medicine: Targeted and Scientific

Modern medicine, a relatively recent development, began to take shape during the Renaissance and grew with the scientific revolution. Discoveries such as microbes, the microscope, and germ theory transformed the understanding of diseases. By the 19th and 20th centuries, modern medicine became highly specialized, emphasizing the diagnosis and treatment of specific symptoms through targeted interventions, often in the form of pharmaceutical drugs.

Modern medicine prioritizes scientific evidence, with drugs developed through rigorous research and clinical trials. Many medications are derived from active plant compounds, synthesized and refined for potency and safety. This approach has led to remarkable advances, particularly in treating acute illnesses and infectious diseases. Here are some of the key differences between the two schools of thought:

Personalization vs. Standardization

- **Herbal Medicine:** Remedies are personalized, considering the individual's constitution, lifestyle, and emotional state. The same condition may be treated differently for each person.
- **Modern Medicine:** Treatment is standardized. Pharmaceuticals are prescribed based on well-defined guidelines, ensuring consistency but often overlooking individual variations.

Complexity vs. Specificity

- **Herbal Medicine:** Remedies often combine multiple herbs for a broader impact, addressing various aspects of health simultaneously.
- **Modern Medicine:** Pharmaceuticals target specific pathways or receptors in the body, making them highly effective for particular conditions but less holistic.

Side Effects and Safety

- **Herbal Medicine:** Generally associated with fewer side effects when used appropriately, but potency can vary, and interactions with medications must be managed carefully.
- **Modern Medicine:** Pharmaceuticals undergo rigorous testing but can have significant side effects, particularly with long-term use.

Preventative vs. Reactive

- **Herbal Medicine:** Emphasizes prevention by maintaining balance and health, often involving long-term lifestyle changes and consistent use of herbs.
- **Modern Medicine:** Primarily reactive, focusing on treating illnesses after they appear; although preventive care is gaining attention.

Natural vs. Synthetic

- **Herbal Medicine:** Uses minimally processed, plant-based ingredients that align with the body's natural processes.
- **Modern Medicine:** Often synthetic, with drugs designed to mimic or enhance natural processes, ensuring purity and potency.

Philosophy of Healing

- **Herbal Medicine:** Believes in the body's natural ability to heal itself, using gentle remedies to restore balance.
- **Modern Medicine:** Focuses on intervention, employing powerful tools like drugs and surgery to directly address disease.

Cost and Accessibility

> ➤ **Herbal Medicine:** Often more affordable and accessible; although sustainably sourced herbs can be costly.
> ➤ **Modern Medicine:** Can be expensive, with advanced treatments and brand-name drugs often out of reach for those without insurance or adequate resources.

From the dawn of human civilization to the rise of modern medicine, herbs have played a central role in the story of healing. Across cultures and centuries, plants have provided not only remedies but also a profound connection to the natural world and to the wisdom of those who came before us. Even as modern medicine transformed healthcare with its precision and speed, the foundational role of herbs remains undeniable—over a quarter of today's pharmaceuticals owe their origins to plants.

Yet, as we marvel at the advancements of science, we risk losing the connection to the plants themselves—their roots in the soil, their role in ecosystems, and the timeless wisdom they carry. As herbalist Jen Bredesen reminds us, there is immense value in working with whole plants rather than isolated chemicals. Herbs not only offer physical healing but also remind us of our shared heritage with the earth, connecting us to the cycles of life that sustain us.

This journey into the origins of herbal medicine lays the groundwork for understanding how we can use herbs effectively today. To truly harness their healing power, it's essential to ensure the quality and integrity of the plants we work with. Whether you're growing your own herbs, sourcing them from trusted suppliers, or crafting remedies, the care and attention you bring to the process can make all the difference.

As we move into Part 2, we'll explore how to source high-quality herbs, grow them ethically, and ensure that the remedies you create are as potent and effective as they are respectful of the natural world. In a world of convenience and shortcuts, reconnecting with the roots of herbalism is not just a choice—it's a commitment to honoring the earth and the traditions that have shaped our understanding of health.

Part 2
THE HERBALIST'S GUIDE

SOURCING ETHICALLY AND GROWING EFFECTIVELY

The potency, safety, and effectiveness of herbal medicines are only as good as the ingredients we use. Whether you're brewing a calming tea or concocting a healing salve, the quality of the herbs you select can make a great difference.

Potency and Effectiveness

The primary reason why high-quality herbs are important is their potency. Potent herbs have a higher concentration of active compounds known as "phytochemicals." In order for the herbs to deliver their desired result, phytochemicals must be present in optimal amounts and balanced proportions. Herbs grown under ideal conditions and harvested at the right time normally have high levels of these crucial compounds.

Safety

Quality also means safety. Herbs not grown, harvested, or stored correctly may contain harmful contaminants such as pesticides, heavy metals, or mold. Such contaminants can not only negate the health benefits but also pose serious health risks to users. That's why it is important to make sure that the herbs you use are sourced from reputable suppliers or grown in controlled environments.

Sustainability

The demand for herbal products has increased in the last few decades. This has caused overharvesting and exploitation of natural resources. High-quality herbs are sourced ethically. This means that the methods used for growing and harvesting support the sustainability of plant species and their natural habitats. This approach helps to maintain ecological balance. It also ensures that these plants can continue to thrive for future generations.

Sensory Quality

The sensory qualities of herbs, especially the flavor, aroma, and color, also indicate their quality. These sensory attributes also are indicative of the herb's freshness. Fresh herbs provide a more pleasant sensory experience, which makes herbal practices more enjoyable.

Tips for Recognizing High-Quality Herbs

You already know why it's important to learn how to pick the best-quality herbs. Therefore, buy good-quality herbs and make sure that you're getting the most out of their natural benefits. Here are some tips for recognizing high-quality herbs and what to look for.

Color and Freshness

One of the first indicators of herb quality is their color. High-quality herbs should display vibrant, natural hues that reflect their freshness and potency. For fresh herbs like basil, the leaves should be bright green and firm. Wilted, yellowing, or spotted leaves are clear signs of poor condition and reduced effectiveness.

Color is equally important for dried herbs. Dried thyme, oregano, or similar herbs should retain their characteristic green or earthy tones. If they appear brown, faded, or dull, it's an indication that the herb has aged and lost some of its potency. Vibrant color is not just aesthetic; it signals the presence of the essential compounds that give herbs their therapeutic properties.

Aroma

Smell is another key indicator of an herb's quality. Fresh herbs should have a strong, distinct aroma that reflects their potency. For instance, rosemary should exude a sharp, pine-like scent, while mint should smell crisp and invigorating. A muted or stale aroma often signals that the herb is past its prime.

Dried herbs, while less aromatic than their fresh counterparts, should still retain a noticeable scent. If a dried herb has little to no fragrance, it likely means the essential oils—the source of its therapeutic properties—have diminished, rendering it less effective.

Taste

Tasting a small piece of an herb can provide valuable insight into its quality. High-quality herbs, whether fresh or dried, should have a robust and distinctive flavor. For example, fresh cilantro should deliver a bold, slightly citrusy taste. If the herb tastes bland or lacks intensity, it's a sign that it may not have been harvested at the right time or stored properly.

The strength of an herb's flavor is directly tied to its phytochemical content—the compounds responsible for its medicinal and culinary properties. A flavorful herb indicates that it still retains the potency needed to be effective in both applications.

Texture

Texture is another reliable indicator of herb quality. Fresh herbs should feel firm and slightly moist to the touch, never wilted or dried out. Their texture reflects their freshness and readiness for use.

For dried herbs, the ideal texture is slightly flexible rather than overly brittle. Properly dried herbs retain a bit of pliability, indicating they were processed and stored correctly. If dried herbs crumble into dust too easily, it's a sign they may have been over-dried or stored for too long, diminishing their potency and effectiveness.

Ethical Sourcing

As discussed in the previous session, high-quality herbs come from ethical and sustainable sources. Ethically sourced herbs are of better quality. And they help preserve plant species and their habitats.

Harvest Time

The timing of an herb's harvest can significantly affect its potency. Every herb has specific growing cycle, picking them at their peak ensures that they have the highest concentration of beneficial compounds. Many herbs are best harvested early in the day, when their essential oils are most concentrated. For example, herbs like lavender and chamomile should be collected in the morning to ensure maximum potency. Always inquire or check if the herbs you're purchasing were harvested at the right time for optimal quality.

Storage and Packaging

Another determinant of quality is how herbs are stored after harvesting. Fresh herbs should be stored in a cool, dry place and kept in a breathable container to prevent mold and rot. Dried herbs should be stored in airtight containers that protect them from light and moisture. Clear packaging is a red flag because exposure to light can degrade the essential oils. Dark, airtight containers are ideal for preserving the quality of dried herbs.

Lack of Contaminates

The purity of herbs is one of the most important aspects of their quality. Herbs should be free from contaminants like pesticides, mold, or heavy metals. To ensure that the herbs you're using are safe, try to purchase from suppliers who follow good manufacturing practices or are certified organic.

Check for Additives and Fillers

When buying packaged or processed herbal products, check the ingredients for any unnecessary additives. Some herbs are sold with added preservatives, dyes, or fillers that dilute their natural effectiveness. Always choose products that are 100% pure herb with no artificial additives.

Reputation of the Supplier

Lastly, the reputation of the supplier or vendor can often tell you a lot about the quality of the herbs they sell. Reputable suppliers normally have strict standards for sourcing, processing, and storing herbs. They may also be transparent about their harvesting methods, ethical sourcing, and whether they test their herbs for purity and contaminants. If you have any doubts, do some research on the supplier and read reviews.

Tips for Sustainable and Ethical Herb Sourcing

As you now know how to identify high-quality herbs, it is time to learn how to source them responsibly for your herbal practice. Here are some practical ways to ensure that you're sourcing herbs sustainably and ethically.

Choose Certified Organic Herbs

Organic certification means that the herbs are grown without synthetic pesticides or fertilizers. These herbs are good for the environment and your health. When you purchase herbs, look for labels like USDA Organic or other recognized organic certifications.

You can also support Fair Trade practices. Fair Trade–certified herbs mean that farmers and workers are paid fairly and work under good conditions. When choosing Fair Trade products, you support communities and promote ethical labor practices.

Opt for Wildcrafted Herbs Carefully

Wildcrafted herbs are gathered from their natural habitats. When you buy wildcrafted herbs, make sure that they are harvested responsibly to prevent overharvesting and damage to ecosystems. Only buy wildcrafted herbs from suppliers who follow sustainable harvesting guidelines.

Grow Your Own Herbs

Starting a small herb garden allows you to control how your herbs are grown. You can use organic methods and ensure that no harmful chemicals are used. Even if you have limited space, you can still grow herbs. Many herbs can be grown in pots on a balcony or windowsill. We'll discuss this more as we move along.

Learn about Endangered Herbs

Some herbs are at risk because of overharvesting and habitat loss. Familiarize yourself with those endangered or threatened plants. For information, check organizations like United Plant Savers. Avoid buying these herbs unless they are cultivated sustainably.

Ask Questions

Don't hesitate to contact suppliers if you have questions about their sourcing practices. Ethical companies will be transparent and willing to share information about how their herbs are grown and harvested.

Reduce Waste

Buy herbs in bulk when possible to reduce packaging waste. Use reusable containers to store your herbs at home.

Support Local Farmers

When you purchase herbs from local farmers' markets, you support your community and reduce the carbon footprint of transporting goods long distances. Also, you can speak directly with the growers about their farming practices.

Educate Yourself

Continuously learn about sustainable practices and stay updated on issues related to herb sourcing. The more you know, the better choices you can make.

Where to Buy Quality Herbs Online

While there are many reputable online sellers, I encourage you to do some research to find the right one for your needs. Below are just a few trusted online sources where you can purchase high-quality herbs.

Mountain Rose Herbs

Mountain Rose Herbs is known for its extensive selection of organic, sustainably sourced herbs. You'll find detailed information about their products online. This company is committed to environmental stewardship. Website: **mountainroseherbs.com**

Frontier Co-op

Frontier Co-op offers a wide range of organic herbs and spices. This company focuses on sustainability and fair trade, which support farmers and communities worldwide. Website: **frontiercoop.com**

Starwest Botanicals

Starwest Botanicals is another good choice for buying organic and wildcrafted herbs. This company emphasizes quality and purity and has certifications for organic and kosher products. Website: **starwest-botanicals.com**

Herb Pharm

Herb Pharm specializes in herbal extracts and tinctures. This company uses organic and sustainably wildcrafted herbs and is transparent about its farming and processing methods. Website: **herb-pharm.com**

Where to Buy Quality Herbs Offline

Local Health Food Stores

Many health food stores carry a selection of bulk herbs. When you shop locally, you can see the products firsthand and ask store staff about their sourcing.

Farmers' Markets

Farmers' markets are excellent places to find fresh, locally grown herbs. You can talk directly with the farmers to learn about their growing practices and perhaps even visit their farms.

Herbalist Shops

Specialty shops that focus on herbal products often have knowledgeable staff who can provide guidance on sourcing and using herbs responsibly.

Community Supported Agriculture (CSA)

If you join a CSA program, you may have access to fresh herbs grown by local farmers. Some CSAs offer herbal shares or include herbs in their regular produce boxes.

Botanical Gardens and Plant Sales

Botanical gardens sometimes host plant sales where you can purchase herb seedlings to grow yourself. This is a great way to source herbs and support educational institutions.

THE IMPORTANCE OF CORRECT DOSAGE

Just like conventional medicine, the effectiveness and safety of herbal remedies depend largely on the correct dosage. If you take too little, it will be ineffective. If you consume too much, you may experience unwanted side effects or even toxicity. For example, excessive usage of potent herbs like comfrey, ephedra, or aconite can have bad side effects. Overdosing can also strain organs like the liver and kidneys, which metabolize and eliminate herbal compounds.

Proper dosage allows the herb to work at its optimal capacity and deliver the therapeutic benefits needed to treat specific conditions.

Factors Influencing Dosage

- **Age:** Children and the elderly may require lower doses due to differences in metabolism and sensitivity.
- **Weight:** Dosage may vary based on body weight. Larger individuals often need higher doses for effectiveness.
- **Overall Health:** People with underlying conditions, especially liver or kidney issues, may need tailored doses to avoid complications.
- **Therapeutic Window:** Each herb has a safe and effective range of dosage. You have to stick to this for proper treatment and to avoid risks.
- **Consistency Matters:** To obtain the most benefits, herbs often require consistent, long-term use at the correct dose, especially in chronic conditions like inflammation or anxiety.
- **Form of Preparation:** Dosages can vary depending on the form of the herb (tinctures, teas, capsules, etc.), because concentrations differ significantly between preparations.
- **Synergistic Effects:** Combining herbs can enhance their healing power but also requires attention to dosage to avoid amplifying side effects or interactions.

It's important that you stick to these guidelines to get the safe and effective outcomes in herbal treatments.

Warning about Herb–Drug Interactions

Just because herbs are natural doesn't mean they are always safe to mix with prescription or over-the-counter drugs. Sometimes, herbs can interfere with medications and cause unwanted or even dangerous effects.

- **Competing Effects:** Some herbs can make medications less effective. For example, St. John's Wort, often used for mood improvement, can reduce the effectiveness of birth control pills, antidepressants, and some heart medications.

- **Increased Potency:** Other herbs can make certain drugs more powerful, which may cause side effects. For example, Ginkgo biloba improves circulation, but it can increase the risk of bleeding if you take blood thinners like aspirin or warfarin.
- **Toxic Reactions:** In some cases, combining herbs with drugs can cause toxicity. Kava, an herb used for anxiety, can worsen liver problems if taken with certain medications that affect liver functions.
- **Timing is Key:** Even if an herb and a drug are safe together, the timing of when you take them can matter. Some herbs might interfere with the way your body absorbs medication, so it's important to space them out.

If you're taking medications, it's always a good idea to talk to a healthcare professional before using herbs.

A doctor or pharmacist can help you avoid harmful interactions and suggest safe herbal alternatives.

Common Risky Combinations:
- Garlic and Ginseng with blood thinners like warfarin (risk of bleeding).
- Echinacea with immunosuppressants (reduces medication effectiveness).
- Licorice Root with blood pressure medications (can cause high blood pressure).

Always look up potential interactions between herbs and medications you're taking. Reliable sources include herbal medicine books, medical websites, and consultations with qualified healthcare providers.

Understanding Your Body's Response to Herbs

Every person's body responds differently to herbs, just like medications or foods. What works well for one person may not work for another.

That's why it's important to pay close attention to how your body reacts to any herb you use.

- **Start slow:** When trying a new herb, start with a smaller dose to see how your body responds before gradually increasing it to the recommended amount. This allows you to monitor for any negative reactions or sensitivities.
- **Listen to your body:** Notice any changes, both positive and negative. Do you feel better or more energized? Does the herb help with your symptoms? Or do you experience any discomfort, upset stomach, or other side effects? If you do, it may be a sign that the herb isn't suitable for you or that the dose needs adjusting.
- **Track your progress:** You may keep a journal of the herbs you use, the doses, and how you feel. This can help you understand which herbs benefit you the most. Tracking your experience also helps to identify patterns over time, such as herbs that may not suit your system.

- ➢ **Consider your unique makeup:** Factors like age, weight, lifestyle, and overall health can all influence how an herb affects you. For instance, someone with a faster metabolism might process herbs more quickly, needing a different dose than someone with a slower metabolism.
- ➢ **Long-term adjustments:** Your body's needs can change over time. What worked for you last year might not have the same effect now. So, it's important to stay aware of how your body continues to react to herbs as you use them.

Some people find that certain forms of herbs—like teas instead of tinctures—work better for their needs. Each body responds differently, so it's worth experimenting with various preparations to discover how you best absorb and benefit from the herb. Let's now explore the different forms of herbal remedies and their best uses.

BEST FORMS FOR HERBAL EFFECTIVENESS

Herbs are most effective when used in the right form because the preparation method plays a critical role in extracting their active compounds. Each method targets different chemical constituents found in herbs, such as alkaloids, tannins, flavonoids, and essential oils. The way these compounds are released depends heavily on the method of extraction and preparation. For example:

- **Water-Based Preparations (Infusions and Decoctions):** These are ideal for extracting water-soluble compounds like tannins and flavonoids. Herbal teas and simmered decoctions are effective for releasing these properties.
- **Alcohol-Based Tinctures:** These excel at pulling out complex or less water-soluble components, such as alkaloids and essential oils, making them a versatile option for many herbs.
- **Oil-Based Infusions:** Oils are perfect for extracting fat-soluble compounds, which makes them ideal for topical applications like salves and balms.

Each herb also has a unique phytochemical profile, meaning certain preparations may be more effective depending on the application. For instance, some herbs work best externally in compresses or poultices, while others are most effective when taken internally. Additionally, combining herbs in specific forms—such as tinctures, capsules, or teas—can create synergistic effects, where the active compounds of one herb enhance the efficacy of another.

The key is to align the preparation method with the herb's chemical properties and the condition being addressed. This approach not only preserves the herb's integrity but also ensures that the body receives the most bioavailable form of its therapeutic compounds.

For practitioners, understanding the nature of each herb and its preparation methods is essential for making informed decisions. This knowledge allows for tailored remedies that maximize the herb's potential and ensure safe, effective treatment.

Infusions

Infusions are used when dealing with the more delicate parts of a plant, such as flowers, leaves, and soft stems. The process is similar to making tea: hot water is poured over the herb; then, it is left to steep for a set period, usually 10–20 minutes. This allows the plant's constituents to infuse into the water.

Herbs like chamomile, peppermint, and lavender respond well to infusions, because their active compounds, including volatile oils and flavonoids, are easily extracted by hot water. Infusions are typically used for soothing, calming, or mildly stimulating remedies and are often drunk for their gentle effects.

How to Make an Infusion:

1. Place 1 to 2 teaspoons of dried herb (or a small handful of fresh herb) into a cup.
2. Pour boiling water over the herb.
3. Cover the cup and let the herb steep for 10–20 minutes.
4. Strain and drink.

Decoctions

This method, on the other hand, is best suited for tougher plant materials like roots, bark, seeds, and berries where the medicinal properties are more tightly bound within the plant. To make a decoction, the herbs are simmered in water for 20–45 minutes. The heat breaks down the cell walls and extracts the deeper compounds (such as alkaloids, glycosides, and other robust phytochemicals).

Herbs like dandelion root, ginger root, and cinnamon bark often require decoctions to release their full medicinal benefits. Decoctions tend to have a stronger, sometimes bitter flavor and are generally used for more potent remedies that often target chronic or deep-seated conditions.

How to Make a Decoction:

1. Place 1 to 2 teaspoons of dried root, bark, or seed into a pot.
2. Add 1–2 cups of cold water.
3. Bring to a boil, then reduce to a simmer for 20–45 minutes.
4. Strain and use as directed, either internally or externally.

Both infusions and decoctions can be adapted for various conditions, and depending on the herbs used, they can support everything from digestive health to immune system function.

Oils

Herbal oils are created by infusing dried or fresh herbs into a carrier oil, such as olive oil, coconut oil, or almond oil. The oil absorbs the herb's active constituents over time, usually through a slow heating process or by allowing the herbs to steep in oil for several weeks. Herbal oils are particularly effective for treating conditions like muscle soreness, joint pain, dry skin, or minor wounds.

Herbs such as calendula, arnica, and St. John's Wort are frequently used in oils for their anti-inflammatory, soothing, and skin-healing properties.

How to Make a Basic Oil:

1. Fill a jar halfway with dried herbs (if using fresh herbs, allow them to wilt for a day to remove excess moisture).

2. Pour a carrier oil over the herbs until fully covered.
3. Seal the jar and let it infuse in a sunny spot for 4–6 weeks, shaking it occasionally.
4. Strain the oil and store in a cool, dark place.

Salves

Salves are made by combining herbal oils with a thickening agent, typically beeswax, to create a semi-solid balm. This form is ideal for targeted, topical applications where the oil alone might be too runny. Salves are often used for skin conditions like rashes, burns, and minor cuts or to relieve muscle aches and joint pain.

By locking the oil in a waxy base, salves stay on the skin longer. This offers prolonged relief and moisture protection.

How to Make a Basic Herbal Salve:

1. Start by creating an herbal oil (as described above).
2. Melt beeswax in a double boiler.
3. Stir the herbal oil into the melted beeswax (a common ratio is 1 ounce of beeswax to 1 cup of oil).
4. Pour the mixture into a jar or tin and let it cool and solidify.

Both oils and salves offer a versatile way to deliver herbal medicine directly to the skin. These formulas provide localized relief with minimal side effects.

Bath Soaks

Herbal bath soaks are a relaxing way to absorb the medicinal benefits of herbs through the skin. When herbs are added to a warm bath, their active compounds are released into the water, and our skin absorbs them. This method combines the soothing effects of a bath with the benefits of herbal therapy. This is quite a popular remedy for certain conditions, such as stress, muscle tension, and skin irritation.

Herbs like lavender, chamomile, and rosemary, and Epsom salts, are frequently used in bath soaks because of their calming and pain-reducing effects. Lavender and chamomile are known as stress relievers, while rosemary is often used to invigorate and soothe sore muscles. Epsom salts, although not an herb, are commonly added to bath soaks for their muscle-relaxing properties due to their magnesium content.

How to Make a Basic Herbal Soak:

1. Combine 1 cup of dried herbs (or a combination of herbs) in a cloth bag or muslin pouch.
2. Fill your bath with warm water.
3. Place the bag in the water and allow it to steep for 10–15 minutes.
4. Get into the bath and soak for 20–30 minutes. Allow your body to absorb the benefits.

Herbal bath soaks are a gentle, noninvasive way to heal physically and mentally. They can easily be customized to individual needs.

Lozenges

Herbal lozenges are a convenient way to ingest herbal medicine, particularly for conditions like soothing sore throats, coughs, and respiratory issues. They are small, dissolvable tablets or candies made from herbal extracts mixed with sugar or honey to form a solid structure that slowly dissolves in the mouth. Lozenges work by allowing the herbs to coat the throat and mouth, which provides localized relief.

Herbs such as slippery elm, marshmallow root, and licorice root are frequently used in lozenges because of their mucilage content, which helps soothe and protect irritated mucous membranes. Other herbs like echinacea, ginger, and thyme may be added for their antimicrobial, anti-inflammatory, and immune-boosting properties. Honey, often used as a base, has its own natural antibacterial and soothing properties.

How to Make a Basic Herbal Lozenge:

1. Brew a strong decoction of herbs by simmering 1–2 tablespoons of dried herbs in 1 cup of water for 20–30 minutes.
2. Strain the liquid and return it to the pot.
3. Add honey or sugar to the liquid and heat gently until it thickens into a syrup-like consistency.
4. Pour the syrup into lozenge molds or onto a parchment-lined baking sheet to form small drops.
5. Let the lozenges cool and harden.

Herbal lozenges are popularly used during cold and flu season. They will give you quick relief from throat irritation.

Steam Inhalations

Herbal steam inhalation is a traditional remedy used to clear congestion, soothe irritated respiratory passages, and improve overall respiratory health. When the steam from boiled herbs is inhaled, the medicinal properties of the herbs are absorbed directly into the respiratory system, where they can work on conditions like colds, sinus infections, and allergies.

Steam helps to moisturize and loosen mucus, while the volatile oils and other compounds in the herbs penetrate deeply into the airways. This reduces inflammation and fights infection. This method is particularly useful for delivering essential oils and other volatile compounds that are easily vaporized by heat.

Herbs like eucalyptus, thyme, peppermint, and rosemary are commonly used in steam inhalation for their ability to open up the airways and provide antimicrobial action. Eucalyptus and peppermint contain high levels of menthol, which has a cooling effect and helps to reduce nasal congestion. Thyme and rosemary, rich in volatile oils, offer strong antibacterial and antiviral properties. They are great choices for respiratory infections.

How to Make a Basic Herbal Steam Inhalation:

1. Bring a pot of water to a boil, then remove it from the heat.
2. Add 1–2 tablespoons of dried herbs (or a few drops of essential oil) to the water.
3. Place a towel over your head and lean over the pot, creating a tent to trap the steam.
4. Inhale deeply through your nose and mouth for 5–10 minutes, taking breaks as needed.

Herbal steam inhalation provides immediate relief for congestion and inflammation. It is especially effective during colds, sinusitis, or seasonal allergies.

Poultices

A poultice is a paste made from fresh or dried herbs that are mashed or ground and applied directly to the skin. Poultices work by delivering the active compounds of the herbs directly to the affected area. They are typically used for drawing out infections, soothing burns, or reducing swelling and pain.

Herbs like comfrey, plantain, and arnica are commonly used in poultices due to their ability to promote tissue regeneration, reduce inflammation, and accelerate healing.

How to Make a Basic Poultice:

1. Crush fresh herbs or rehydrate dried herbs by soaking them in hot water until they form a paste.
2. Apply the herb paste directly to the skin or onto a clean cloth, then place it on the affected area.
3. Cover the poultice with a bandage or wrap and leave it in place for 1–2 hours, or as needed.

Compresses

A compress is made by soaking a cloth in an herbal infusion or decoction and applying it to the skin. Similar to poultices, compresses are less messy and more practical for larger areas or situations where a direct application of herbs is not feasible. They can effectively reduce muscle tension, soothe sprains, and treat skin irritations or infections. Herbs like chamomile, calendula, and witch hazel are commonly used in compresses for their anti-inflammatory, astringent, and soothing properties.

How to Make a Basic Herbal Compress:

1. Brew a strong infusion or decoction of herbs.
2. Soak a clean cloth or bandage in the liquid and wring out the excess.
3. Apply the cloth to the affected area, securing it in place with a bandage if needed.
4. Leave the compress on for 15–30 minutes, reapplying as necessary.

When I first started exploring the world of herbs, I was overwhelmed by the sheer number of choices. It felt like stepping into a vast forest where every plant whispered a secret, and I didn't know which ones to trust. So, I decided to start small, with the herbs that felt approachable and familiar—the kind my grandmother used to grow in her kitchen garden.

Those first few plants became my teachers. They were forgiving, resilient, and full of wisdom. Each leaf I harvested and each mistake I made deepened my understanding and connection to the natural world.

The next chapter introduces 10 sacred and remarkably beginner-friendly herbs—plants that have stood the test of time in their simplicity and power. These herbs are perfect for those just starting their journey into herbalism and are easy to grow, use, and love. Let's discover why they've been cherished for generations and how they can become a part of your life, too.

HERBAL REMEDY VIDEO TUTORIALS BELOW!

Hi there! It's Ava, and I'm thrilled you're exploring my home apothecary book. How are you finding the recipes and remedies? I hope they're inspiring you as much as they've rejuvenated my life and health!

Experience Herbalism Like Never Before:

I understand that sometimes reading about processes isn't quite the same as seeing them in action. That's why I've put together an exclusive video playlist just for you! Over the past decade, I've captured my herbalism journey in detail, and these videos are packed with hands-on demonstrations to enhance your learning and skills.

Here is a small portion of what is in the playlist:

- **Tinctures:** Expert extraction methods revealed.
- **Compresses:** Natural solutions for pain and wound care.
- **Salves:** Simple recipes for skin and body healing.
- **Steam Inhalations:** Effective techniques for respiratory health.
- **Lozenges:** Easy-to-make remedies for throat relief.
- **More Insights:** Dive into additional herbal practices.

bit.ly/homeapothecary2025

Why Watch the Videos?

- **Practical Demonstrations:** See the textures, colors, and techniques in real time—perfect for visual learners.
- **Detailed Explanations:** Understand the 'why' behind each method, enhancing your ability to replicate and adapt recipes.
- **Personal Touch:** Feel connected as I share personal tips and stories from many years of experience.

Get Started Now!

Get comfortable, set up your herbal workstation, and start watching today to bring the power of nature right into your home! Scan the QR code or use the link to start watching today.

Happy Healing,

Ava

THE HERBAL INITIATION: 10 SACRED STARTER HERBS FOR BEGINNERS

When I first started learning about herbalism, I didn't begin with rare or exotic plants. I started small, with the same herbs that grew in my grandmother's backyard. Her garden wasn't fancy, but it was alive—mint along the path, chamomile by the fence, and lemon balm in the corner, humming with bees. She taught me that herbalism isn't about mastering hundreds of plants at once; it's about building a relationship with a few trusted allies.

I remember the way she handled those plants—with care, as if they were old friends. She showed me how to pinch off mint leaves to release their invigorating scent and steep chamomile flowers for a tea that felt like a warm hug. Each herb had a purpose and a lesson to teach.

"Start with what you know," she would say as she planted seeds, her hands brushing the soil. "Watch how they grow, how they smell, how they change with the seasons. They'll show you what they're good for."

So, I did. Mint eased my stomach, chamomile calmed my restless mind, and lemon balm soothed my stress. Slowly, I realized herbalism wasn't just about remedies—it was about connection. These plants weren't tools; they were allies, rooted in tradition and wisdom.

Every herbal journey should begin with the basics—herbs that are easy to grow, safe to use, and endlessly versatile. They may be humble, but they're powerful in their simplicity. In this chapter, I'll introduce you to ten beginner-friendly herbs, each one a gentle guide to the world of herbal healing. Let's start with these trusted friends and see where the journey takes us.

CHAMOMILE (MATRICARIA CHAMOMILLA)

Chamomile, a small yet mighty herb, is part of the daisy family. This herb is known for its delicate, white-petaled flowers that cradle a golden center. Native to Europe and Western Asia, this gentle healer has been cherished for centuries for its medicinal properties.

Historical Context

Chamomile has roots into ancient civilizations. The Egyptians, Greeks, and Romans held it in high regard, especially for its ability to ease digestive woes and calm the nerves. It was used in sacred rituals, brewed into teas, and even applied as a natural cosmetic by noblewomen. Over time, its reputation as a universal healer spread across continents.

Active Compounds and Benefits

Chamomile's power comes from its rich profile of active compounds, particularly apigenin, a flavonoid that imparts many of its therapeutic properties.

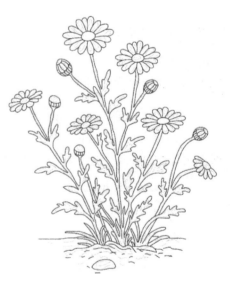

- **Calming and Sedative:** Chamomile is famed for its calming effects, often used to ease anxiety, stress, and insomnia.
- **Digestive Aid:** It soothes the stomach, relieves indigestion, gas, and colic.
- **Anti-inflammatory:** Chamomile helps reduce inflammation, both internally and externally, and is a popular remedy for skin irritations like eczema and rashes.

Most Potent Method of Ingestion

Chamomile's most potent form is as a tea or infusion. Steeping its dried flowers releases apigenin, making it a gentle but powerful ally for both the mind and body. Chamomile tinctures and extracts are also effective, especially for those seeking quick relief from stress or sleep disturbances. Combining chamomile, lemon balm, and lavender in an herbal tea creates a deeply soothing blend that calms the mind, relaxes the body, and prepares you for a peaceful night's rest.

Simple Recipe: Chamomile Tea

Add 1–2 teaspoons of dried chamomile flowers, 1 cup of hot water. Steep chamomile flowers in hot water for 5–10 minutes. Strain and enjoy a calming cup of tea, particularly before bed for restful sleep.

PEPPERMINT (MENTHA PIPERITA)

Peppermint, with its refreshing scent and cool flavor, is a hybrid of watermint and spearmint. Its vibrant green leaves and invigorating aroma make it a favorite in both kitchens and herbal medicine cabinets. It is native to Europe and the Middle East.

Historical Context

Peppermint has been revered for its medicinal properties for over 3,000 years, dating back to the ancient Egyptians. It was widely used by the Greeks and Romans as a digestive aid, and it continues to be a popular herb in traditional remedies worldwide. Throughout history, peppermint has also been used to freshen the air, cleanse the spirit, and purify the body.

Active Compounds and Benefits

Peppermint owes much of its potency to menthol, the compound responsible for its cooling, soothing sensation.

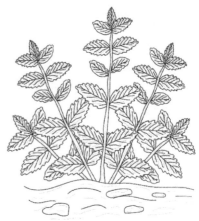

- **Digestive Relief:** Peppermint helps relieve indigestion, bloating, and gas by relaxing the muscles of the digestive tract.
- **Headache and Pain Relief:** Its cooling properties make it effective for soothing headaches and muscle pain when applied topically as an oil or balm.
- **Respiratory Support:** Menthol can clear nasal congestion, making peppermint a popular remedy for colds and coughs.

Most Potent Method of Ingestion

Peppermint tea is a time-honored way to enjoy its digestive benefits. Peppermint essential oil, when diluted and applied topically, is highly potent for treating headaches or sore muscles. Its aroma, whether from fresh leaves or essential oil, also brings mental clarity and refreshment.

A combination of peppermint, ginger, and fennel makes a soothing tea for digestive issues, each herb enhancing the other's ability to calm and balance the gut.

Simple Recipe: Peppermint Tea for Digestion

Add 1 teaspoon of dried peppermint leaves to 1 cup of boiling water. Steep the peppermint leaves in hot water for 5–7 minutes. Sip slowly to soothe an upset stomach or aid digestion after meals.

LAVENDER (LAVANDULA ANGUSTIFOLIA)

Lavender, with its fragrant purple blossoms, is a timeless symbol of peace and tranquility. Native to the Mediterranean, its elegant flowers have perfumed the air and healed the body for thousands of years.

Historical Context

Lavender has been a beloved herb since ancient times, particularly among the Greeks and Romans who used it to scent their baths, soothe their skin, and calm their minds. In medieval Europe, lavender was placed under pillows to invite restful sleep and ward off evil spirits. Over the centuries, it has been cherished not only for its beauty but also for its profound ability to heal the body and mind.

Active Compounds and Benefits

The magic of lavender lies in its essential oil, particularly the compound linalool, which gives it its characteristic calming and healing effects.

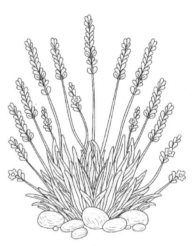

- **Calming and Sedative:** Lavender is renowned for its ability to ease anxiety, promote relaxation, and combat insomnia.
- **Skin Healing:** Its antiseptic and anti-inflammatory properties make lavender an effective remedy for burns, wounds, and skin irritations.
- **Headache and Muscle Pain Relief:** Lavender's soothing effects can help alleviate tension headaches and muscle aches when applied as an oil or balm.

Most Potent Method of Ingestion

Lavender's most potent form is as an essential oil. A few drops in a diffuser can calm the mind, while diluted oil applied to the skin soothes aches and pains. Lavender tea is also effective for reducing stress and inducing relaxation. A blend of lavender, rosemary, and chamomile creates a powerful, fragrant tea that promotes peace of mind, eases headaches, and encourages restful sleep.

Simple Recipe: Lavender Bath Soak

Add half a cup of dried lavender flowers and 1 cup Epsom salts into a warm bath. Soak for 20 minutes to relax muscles and relieve stress.

LEMON BALM (MELISSA OFFICINALIS)

Historical Context

Lemon balm has been treasured since the Middle Ages. It was known as "the elixir of life" for its ability to uplift the spirit. Its use dates back to ancient Greece and Rome, where it was favored for its calming and mood-enhancing properties. In medieval times, it was often used to ease depression and anxiety.

Active Compounds and Benefits

Lemon balm is rich in rosmarinic acid and flavonoids, which contribute to its powerful effects.

- **Stress Relief:** Its calming properties help ease anxiety and restlessness, promoting relaxation and improving sleep quality.
- **Digestive Aid:** Lemon balm soothes the stomach, relieves bloating, and helps with indigestion.
- **Antiviral:** Its antiviral effects, particularly against cold sores, make it a good natural skincare.

Most Potent Method of Ingestion

Lemon balm works best as a tea or tincture to calm the nervous system and support digestion. For skin applications, a salve or infused oil can be used to soothe cold sores and other irritations. In aromatherapy, its refreshing, lemony scent helps ease tension.

Simple Recipe: Lemon Balm Infusion

Add 1 tablespoon of dried lemon balm leaves to 1 cup of hot water. Steep the lemon balm leaves in hot water for 10 minutes. Strain and drink to reduce anxiety or stress.

GINGER (ZINGIBER OFFICINALE)

Historical Context

Ginger has been a cornerstone of traditional medicine in Asia and the Middle East for over 5,000 years. In Ayurvedic and Chinese medicine, it is commonly used to boost digestion, treat nausea, and increase vitality. Today, it remains a global favorite for its warming and healing properties.

Active Compounds and Benefits

Ginger's medicinal power comes from gingerol, a potent bioactive compound.

- **Digestive Booster:** Ginger stimulates digestion, eases nausea, and reduces bloating.
- **Anti-inflammatory:** Gingerol has strong anti-inflammatory effects and is helpful for arthritis and muscle pain.
- **Immune Support:** Its warming properties and antioxidants help fight colds and boost the immune system.

Most Potent Method of Ingestion

Ginger, when taken as a fresh or dried tea, provides warmth and relief from nausea or digestive issues. Ginger tinctures and powders are excellent for daily use, while fresh ginger can be added to food for both flavor and health benefits. A poultice of ginger can also soothe muscle pain or joint stiffness.

Simple Recipe: Ginger Honey Syrup

Add 1 tablespoon fresh ginger (grated) to 1 cup water. Simmer ginger in water for 10–15 minutes. Strain and mix in honey. Take 1–2 teaspoons as needed for digestive relief or nausea.

CALENDULA (CALENDULA OFFICINALIS)

Historical Context

Calendula, also known as "common marigold" (not to be confused with the *Tagetes* marigold), has been used for centuries by cultures across Europe and the Mediterranean. In ancient Rome, it was cherished for its wound-healing and skin-soothing abilities. Medieval herbalists prized it for treating infections and inflammation.

Active Compounds and Benefits

Calendula is packed with carotenoids and flavonoids, which are responsible for its vibrant color and healing power.

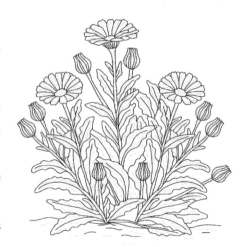

- ➤ **Skin Healing:** Calendula's anti-inflammatory and antiseptic properties make it ideal for treating minor wounds, burns, and skin irritations.
- ➤ **Anti-inflammatory:** Reduces swelling and promotes tissue regeneration, especially for eczema and dermatitis.
- ➤ **Antifungal:** Helps treat fungal infections, including athlete's foot and yeast infections.

Most Potent Method of Ingestion

Calendula is most potent when applied topically as a salve or infused oil, which makes it a go-to for wound care and skin irritations. It can also be brewed into a tea or tincture for its anti-inflammatory benefits, particularly for internal inflammation and digestive discomfort. Its flowers are often infused into oils for gentle skincare solutions.

Simple Recipe: Calendula Salve

Add half a cup of dried calendula flowers to half a cup of olive oil. Infuse the calendula flowers in olive oil for several hours over low heat. Strain, then mix with a quarter cup of melted beeswax to create a healing salve for skin irritations.

HERBS FOR DIGESTIVE ISSUES

THYME (THYMUS VULGARIS)

Historical Context

Thyme has been cherished since ancient times, from the Egyptians who used it in embalming to the Greeks who burned it as incense for courage. In the Middle Ages, it was gifted to knights for bravery and was a staple in medicinal gardens for treating respiratory issues and infections.

Active Compounds and Benefits

Thyme is rich in thymol, a powerful compound known for its antiseptic and antimicrobial properties.

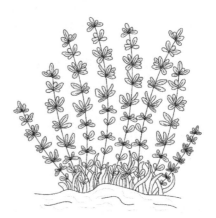

- ➤ **Respiratory Support:** Helps relieve coughs, bronchitis, and congestion by loosening phlegm and soothing the airways.
- ➤ **Antiseptic:** Its strong antibacterial properties make it effective for cleaning wounds and fighting infections.
- ➤ **Digestive Aid:** Eases indigestion and reduces bloating, making it a trusted herb for overall digestive health.

Most Potent Method of Ingestion

Thyme tea or syrup is ideal for soothing coughs and clearing respiratory passages. A steam inhalation using thyme essential oil is also beneficial for congestion. For topical use, thyme-infused oils or salves can be applied to cuts and scrapes to promote healing.

Simple Recipe: Thyme Steam Inhalation

Add 1–2 teaspoons dried thyme to 1 bowl of boiling water. Place a towel over your head and inhale the steam for 5–10 minutes to help relieve congestion or respiratory issues.

ECHINACEA (ECHINACEA PURPUREA)

Historical Context

Native to North America, Echinacea has long been revered by Indigenous peoples for its immune-boosting and wound-healing abilities. It became widely popular during the 19th century, particularly in Western herbalism, as a treatment for infections, colds, and flu.

Active Compounds and Benefits

Echinacea contains a wealth of bioactive compounds, including alkamides, phenolic acids, and polysaccharides.

- **Immune Booster:** Stimulates the immune system, which makes it highly effective in fighting off colds, flu, and other infections.
- **Anti-inflammatory:** Reduces inflammation and supports faster recovery from infections and injuries.
- **Antiviral:** Helps fend off viral infections, particularly in the early stages of illness.

Most Potent Method of Ingestion

Echinacea works best as a tincture or tea to strengthen the immune system, especially at the first sign of a cold. It can also be used in capsules for daily immune support. Topically, echinacea-infused salves aid in wound healing and reducing inflammation from insect bites or skin irritations.

Simple Recipe: Echinacea Immune Boosting Tea

Add 1 teaspoon of dried echinacea root, to 1 cup of boiling water. Steep echinacea root in hot water for 10–15 minutes. Strain and drink during cold and flu season to help boost immunity.

HERBS FOR DIGESTIVE ISSUES

ROSEMARY (ROSMARINUS OFFICINALIS)

Historical Context

Rosemary has been an essential herb in the Mediterranean for thousands of years, revered for its memory-enhancing properties. Ancient Greeks and Romans believed it could strengthen the mind, and it was often worn as a symbol of remembrance. It has also been used for its uplifting and protective qualities.

Active Compounds and Benefits

Rosemary is packed with rosmarinic acid and essential oils like cineole and camphor.

- **Cognitive Support:** Rosemary improves memory and concentration, which makes it a natural brain tonic.
- **Antioxidant:** It protects the body from oxidative stress, supporting overall health and longevity.
- **Circulation Booster:** Its warming properties stimulate blood flow, easing muscle pain and tension.

Most Potent Method of Ingestion

Rosemary tea or tincture is ideal for enhancing memory and mental clarity. A rosemary-infused oil or balm can be applied topically to relieve sore muscles and improve circulation. Rosemary essential oil, inhaled or diffused, can also uplift the mood and energize the mind.

Simple Recipe: Rosemary Hair Rinse

Add 1 tablespoon of dried rosemary to 1 cup of boiling water. Steep the rosemary in hot water for 15 minutes, strain, and use the cooled liquid as a hair rinse to stimulate scalp health and shine.

DANDELION (TARAXACUM OFFICINALE)

Historical Context

Often seen as a pesky weed, dandelion has actually been treasured for centuries for its medicinal value. Ancient Egyptians, Greeks, and Romans used it for its diuretic and digestive properties. In traditional Chinese and Native American medicine, dandelion was prized as a tonic for the liver and kidneys.

Active Compounds and Benefits

Dandelion is rich in vitamins A, C, and K, and minerals like iron and potassium, but it's the bitter compounds, taraxacin and inulin, that give it its powerful healing properties.

- **Liver Detoxifier:** Dandelion supports liver function by promoting the production of bile, aiding digestion, and flushing toxins.
- **Diuretic:** It acts as a natural diuretic, helping reduce water retention and purify the body.
- **Digestive Aid:** It relieves constipation and encourages a healthy gut by stimulating digestive juices.

Most Potent Method of Ingestion

Dandelion root tea or tincture is the most potent way to support liver health and digestion. The leaves, when consumed fresh in salads or brewed as a tea, offer excellent diuretic benefits. Dandelion root can also be roasted and used as a caffeine-free coffee substitute, providing gentle digestive support while detoxifying the liver.

Simple Recipe: Dandelion Root Tea

Add 1 teaspoon of dried dandelion root, to 1 cup of hot water. Simmer the dandelion root in hot water for 10–15 minutes. Strain and drink to support liver function and digestion.

THE HERBAL INITIATION: SIMPLE YET POWERFUL BEGINNINGS

As you start preparing herbal remedies by yourself, remember that even the most basic preparations can have a profound impact. Some of the world's most cherished remedies are created with simple ingredients. A soothing cup of chamomile tea or a lavender salve for sore muscles may seem modest, but their healing power is real and time-tested.

To make a difference in your own well-being, you don't need complicated formulas or rare herbs. The beauty of herbalism lies in its accessibility—using nature's gifts in a way that fits seamlessly into everyday life. Whether you're brewing a tea, making an infusion, or preparing a balm, the process itself is healing. When you work with herbs, you connect to the earth and to your body's own innate ability to restore balance.

Mastery comes with practice, so don't feel overwhelmed by the idea of having to know every herb or technique. Begin small. Pick one or two herbs to work with at first and experiment with simple recipes. Over time, you'll start to develop a deeper understanding of how different herbs work, both individually and in combination.

Each new preparation will be another step in your growing knowledge and confidence. Therefore, start with these sacred 10 herbs, and from there, let curiosity guide you. Remember that herbalism is a lifelong practice; your journey has just begun, and the possibilities are endless.

PART 3
EXPANDING YOUR HERBAL KNOWLEDGE: ADDRESSING SPECIFIC AILMENTS

In the previous chapter, we explored 10 foundational herbs to begin your journey into herbalism. Now, we'll dive deeper, expanding our focus to 201 medicinal herbs, each carefully selected for its versatility and effectiveness in supporting various aspects of health—from digestion and skincare to immune function and mental well-being.

As I ventured beyond the foundational herbs, I discovered plants like calendula and ashwagandha—herbs I'd never encountered before but that quickly became staples in my practice. Calendula revealed the soothing power of flowers, while ashwagandha demonstrated how deeply plants can support both mind and body during times of stress. Each new herb brought fresh insights and strengthened my connection to nature's incredible healing potential.

In this chapter, each herb is presented with its historical context, active compounds, and key benefits. You'll learn about the most effective ways to use each herb, along with a simple recipe to address specific conditions. Additionally, I'll introduce an "ally herb" for each plant—a complementary herb that enhances its potency when combined.

Together, these tools will help you not only expand your herbal knowledge but also apply it practically to create powerful remedies for both common ailments and more complex health challenges.

HERBS FOR
DIGESTIVE ISSUES

SOOTHING DIGESTIVE TRACT INFLAMMATION

1. Slippery Elm (*Ulmus rubra*)

Historical Context

Long cherished by Native American tribes, slippery elm was revered for its ability to heal and soothe. Its bark, often stripped from elm trees in the height of spring, was traditionally used to treat wounds, sore throats, and digestive complaints. During the harshest winters, it even served as a nutritious survival food. Slippery elm was used for centuries as a remedy for inflammation and irritation, especially within the digestive system.

Active Compounds and Their Benefits

Slippery elm's magic lies in its mucilage—a gel-like substance that forms when mixed with water. This mucilage coats and protects inflamed tissues, creating a protective barrier that soothes and heals. Rich in tannins and polysaccharides, slippery elm calms irritation and encourages tissue regeneration. Reducing inflammation along the digestive tract helps with conditions like gastritis, ulcerative colitis, and acid reflux.

Most Potent Method of Ingestion

A warm infusion is the most potent way to harness slippery elm's soothing properties. The mucilage forms when the powdered inner bark is steeped in hot water. This creates a smooth, comforting gel that lines the stomach and intestines, which allows immediate relief from inflammation and irritation.

Simple Recipe: Slippery Elm Infusion

Add 1 teaspoon of powdered slippery elm bark to 1 cup of hot water. Mix the powdered bark with hot water and stir well. Let it sit for a few minutes to thicken. Sip slowly to soothe the digestive tract.

Best Herbs to Use Together

Combine slippery elm with marshmallow root for enhanced mucilage and digestive support. A dash of licorice root adds anti-inflammatory power, making this blend especially useful for calming irritated tissues and promoting healing.

2. Licorice Root (*Glycyrrhiza glabra*)

Historical Context

For over 4,000 years, licorice root has been honored in traditional medicine systems from ancient Egypt to China. Known as "the great harmonizer," in traditional Chinese medicine, licorice is used to bring balance to herbal formulas. The Greeks and Romans used it to ease coughs and soothe stomach ailments. Its sweet flavor, hiding beneath earthy notes, has earned it a reputation both as a medicinal herb and a flavoring agent in candies. Yet, beyond its taste lies healing properties, particularly for inflamed and irritated digestive linings.

Active Compounds and Their Benefits

The key active component in licorice root is glycyrrhizin, a compound with potent anti-inflammatory and soothing effects. Glycyrrhizin helps calm irritation in the digestive tract by forming a protective coating over the mucous membranes. This makes it highly effective for conditions like gastritis, peptic ulcers, and acid reflux. Additionally, licorice has antioxidant and antimicrobial properties, further contributing to its healing potential.

Most Potent Method of Ingestion

Licorice root is most potent when taken as a decoction or tincture. A decoction, where the root is gently simmered in water, extracts the beneficial compounds and creates a soothing drink for irritated digestive tissues. Alternatively, a tincture offers a concentrated dose that can be taken before meals to help calm inflammation and support overall digestive health.

Simple Recipe: Licorice Root Decoction

Add 1 tablespoon of dried licorice root to 2 cups of water. Simmer the licorice root in water for 10–15 minutes. Strain and drink warm to soothe inflammation in the digestive tract.

Best Herbs to Use Together

Licorice root pairs beautifully with chamomile for calming both the digestive system and the mind. Combine it with slippery elm for enhanced mucilage and soothing effects on the digestive tract.

STIMULATING DIGESTION

3. Gentian Root (*Gentiana lutea*)

Historical Context

Deep within the towering mountains of Europe, gentian root has been cherished since ancient times for its potent bitter flavor and digestive benefits. It was named after King Gentius of Illyria, who is said to have first discovered its medicinal properties in the second century BCE. In traditional European herbalism, gentian root was employed as a remedy for indigestion, fevers, and even snake bites. Its status as a digestive tonic carried through medieval apothecaries, where it was used to restore vitality to the weak and sluggish after heavy feasts.

Active Compounds and Their Benefits

Gentian's magic lies in its potent bitter compounds—gentiopicroside, amarogentin, and swertiamarin—each working in harmony to ignite the digestive fires. These bitter compounds stimulate the taste receptors, sending signals to the brain to kickstart the digestive system. The stomach releases more acid and enzymes, while the liver produces bile, all in perfect unison to break down food more efficiently. Gentian root is particularly beneficial for those with sluggish digestion, weak appetite, or low stomach acid.

Most Potent Method of Ingestion

A tincture is the most potent way to harness gentian root's powers. When taken 10–15 minutes before meals, it primes the digestive system, making it easier to process food. Gentian tinctures can also be added to a small glass of water to dilute the intensity of their bitterness.

Simple Recipe: Gentian Digestive Tincture

Place 1 tablespoon of gentian root in a jar, covering it with a cup of vodka or brandy. Let it sit for 4–6 weeks, shaking occasionally. Strain the tincture into a dark glass bottle and take 10–15 drops before meals.

Best Herbs to Use Together

Combine gentian root with warming herbs like fennel and ginger for enhanced digestion, or blend it with dandelion root to create a comprehensive liver tonic.

4. Artichoke Leaf (*Cynara scolymus*)

Historical Context

The artichoke, a regal plant with ties to the Mediterranean's rich cultural history, has long been famous for culinary and medicinal uses. The ancient Greeks and Romans celebrated it as a delicacy and a remedy. Known to stimulate bile production, it was used to aid digestion, particularly of rich and fatty foods. Artichoke's reputation persisted through the ages, particularly in Renaissance Europe, where it was enjoyed by royalty not just for its taste but for its ability to soothe overindulgence and promote liver health.

Active Compounds and Their Benefits

The primary healing compounds found in artichoke leaf are cynarin and luteolin. Cynarin, a unique bitter compound, stimulates bile production, improving fat digestion and reducing bloating. Thanks to luteolin, artichoke's antioxidant properties help protect the liver from damage and reduce inflammation in the digestive tract. By promoting healthy bile flow, artichoke leaf aids the body in processing heavy, greasy meals and can be a helpful ally for those suffering from indigestion, gas, or sluggish digestion.

Most Potent Method of Ingestion

A tincture made from artichoke leaf is the most potent way to harness its bile-stimulating powers, particularly when taken before meals. However, an infusion (tea) is a gentler method that can be sipped after meals to encourage digestion. Those with sluggish bile flow or fat malabsorption may find more immediate relief from the tincture's concentrated form.

Simple Recipe: Artichoke Leaf Tea

Add 1 teaspoon of dried artichoke leaf to 1 cup of boiling water. Steep the artichoke leaf in boiling water for 10–15 minutes, then strain. Drink before or after meals to support digestion, particularly when eating heavier foods.

Best Herbs to Use Together

Pair artichoke leaf with milk thistle and dandelion for a complete liver and digestive tonic, or combine it with warming herbs like ginger or cardamom for additional digestive support.

RELIEVING BLOATING AND GAS

5. Caraway (*Carum carvi*)

Historical Context

Caraway has long been known for its digestive healing powers. The ancient Egyptians buried it with their dead, believing in its protective qualities, while the Romans celebrated it as a culinary and medicinal treasure. In medieval Europe, caraway seeds were used in bread to ward off witches and evil spirits, but more commonly, they were known to soothe bloated bellies and ease digestion after hearty meals. The seeds of *Carum carvi* have been woven into folklore and medicine alike, cherished across cultures for their ability to calm turbulent digestion.

Active Compounds and Their Benefits

Caraway seeds contain compounds like carvone, limonene, and anethole. These active compounds help relax the muscles of the digestive tract, allowing trapped gas to be released and bloating to be alleviated. Carvone, the most prominent, is particularly known for stimulating digestive secretions and reducing painful spasms in the gut. Caraway also encourages the smooth passage of food through the intestines, which prevents stagnation that can lead to gas buildup. Its mild antimicrobial properties can help balance gut flora, further supporting healthy digestion.

Most Potent Method of Ingestion

Caraway seeds are best consumed as an infusion (tea) or simply chewed after meals. The warmth of a tea extracts the volatile oils and ensures gentle but powerful relief from bloating and gas. However, the seeds can also be included in food to prevent bloating, making it a functional and flavorful remedy.

Simple Recipe: Caraway Tea for Bloating

Add 1 teaspoon of crushed caraway seeds to 1 cup of boiling water. Steep the crushed seeds in boiling water for 10 minutes. Strain, and sip slowly after meals to ease bloating and gas.

Best Herbs to Use Together

For enhanced digestive relief, combine caraway with fennel or ginger, both of which have strong carminative properties. Caraway also pairs well with peppermint to soothe digestive spasms.

6. Anise (*Pimpinella anisum*)

Historical Context

The aromatic sweetness of anise has enchanted civilizations for millennia. Ancient Egyptians, Greeks, and Romans used this herb not only as a flavoring in food and drink but also as an ally in treating digestive woes. Roman legionnaires consumed anise to ease bloating after feasts, while in medieval Europe, it was commonly chewed to freshen breath and settle the stomach. Its star-shaped seeds, often mistaken for those of its cousin star anise, are still popular in digestive tonics and after-dinner treats.

Active Compounds and Their Benefits

The magic of anise lies in its volatile oils, primarily anethole, estragole, and limonene. These compounds work synergistically to relax the digestive tract, reducing cramping and allowing trapped gas to be released. Anethole, the main compound, is a powerful carminative, meaning it prevents the formation of gas in the gastrointestinal tract while soothing inflammation. Anise also stimulates the secretion of digestive enzymes, helping to break down food more efficiently and prevent bloating.

Most Potent Method of Ingestion

Anise is best enjoyed as a tea or tincture, but chewing the seeds after meals also provides immediate relief. Anise tea is gentle enough for regular use and is especially effective when sipped after heavy, rich meals. The warmth helps extract the volatile oils, which maximizes their carminative benefits.

Simple Recipe: Anise Digestive Tea

Add 1 teaspoon of crushed anise seeds to 1 cup of boiling water. Steep the crushed seeds in boiling water for 10 minutes. Strain and drink after meals to relieve bloating and gas.

Best Herbs to Use Together

Anise pairs beautifully with fennel and peppermint for a comprehensive digestive tonic. It also blends well with chamomile, creating a soothing tea that calms both the stomach and the nerves.

NAUSEA AND VOMITING RELIEF

7. Meadowsweet (*Filipendula ulmaria*)

Historical Context

Known as the "Queen of the Meadow," meadowsweet has been used for centuries for its medicinal qualities. The Druids of ancient Celtic cultures considered it one of their sacred herbs, while in medieval Europe, it was prized as a remedy for fevers and stomach ailments. The herb also played a part in the development of aspirin, with its active compounds inspiring the creation of the modern pain reliever. Yet meadowsweet's soft fragrance and gentle healing power have made it more than just a remedy for pain—it is a balm for queasy stomachs and unsettled digestion.

Active Compounds and Their Benefits

Meadowsweet is rich in salicylates, flavonoids, and tannins, which combine to provide potent anti-inflammatory, soothing, and astringent effects. The herb contains salicin, a precursor to salicylic acid (found in aspirin), which helps reduce nausea and vomiting by calming inflammation in the stomach lining. Its tannins also work as a mild astringent, tightening irritated tissues and reducing digestive upset. Flavonoids in meadowsweet protect the gastrointestinal tract from irritation, making it particularly helpful in soothing nausea and easing discomfort.

Most Potent Method of Ingestion

Meadowsweet is often used as a tincture or capsule to relieve nausea quickly and efficiently. Tinctures are particularly powerful due to their ability to be absorbed rapidly, offering near-immediate relief. A poultice made from meadowsweet can also be applied over the stomach to calm digestive spasms.

Simple Recipe: Meadowsweet Tincture

Place 1 ounce of dried meadowsweet in a glass jar and cover with 4 ounces of alcohol (vodka or brandy). Seal tightly and store in a cool, dark place for 4–6 weeks, shaking occasionally. Strain and store the tincture in a dark glass bottle. Take 15–30 drops in water when nausea strikes.

Best Herbs to Use Together

Meadowsweet pairs beautifully with ginger or peppermint, both known for their ability to calm nausea. Chamomile can also complement its soothing properties for added digestive relief.

8. Catnip (*Nepeta cataria*)

Historical Context

Famous for its intoxicating effect on cats, catnip (also known as "catmint") has a much gentler reputation in human medicine. Its use as a remedy dates back to Roman times, when it was relied upon to ease nervous tension and stomach ailments. In medieval Europe, catnip tea was a popular folk remedy for fevers and digestive woes. Although its name suggests it's only for felines, catnip is effective for calming digestive upset in humans and is often served as soothing teas or tinctures.

Active Compounds and Their Benefits

Catnip contains volatile oils, including nepetalactone, thymol, and carvacrol, which provide calming effects. Nepetalactone, the compound that drives cats wild, also works on humans by relaxing smooth muscles, particularly in the digestive tract. This makes it effective in easing nausea, vomiting, and indigestion. Catnip's mild sedative qualities also help relieve anxiety-induced nausea, allowing the body to relax and the digestive system to settle. The herb's antispasmodic and carminative properties work in harmony to soothe the stomach lining and reduce nausea.

Most Potent Method of Ingestion

Catnip works beautifully as a tincture or steam inhalation to alleviate nausea quickly. A tincture can be taken in small doses when nausea arises, while a steam inhalation made with fresh catnip leaves offers immediate relief for queasiness, especially when associated with colds or flu.

Simple Recipe: Catnip Steam Inhalation

Place a handful of fresh catnip leaves in a bowl and pour boiling water over them. Lean over the bowl, cover your head with a towel to trap the steam, and breathe deeply for 5–10 minutes. The calming aroma helps reduce nausea and digestive discomfort.

Best Herbs to Use Together

Catnip pairs well with lemon balm or chamomile, both of which enhance its calming properties. Combined with fennel, it can also help alleviate gas and bloating, making it a comprehensive digestive remedy.

BALANCING GUT FLORA

9. Garlic (*Allium sativum*)

Historical Context

In ancient Egypt, Greece, and China, garlic was well known for its medicinal properties for thousands of years. Greek athletes consumed it to enhance strength and endurance, while Egyptian laborers used it to boost their immunity. Its use in folk medicine is nearly universal, known for its potent ability to combat infections and balance the body's internal systems. Garlic has always been more than a spice. It's a symbol of health, strength, and protection. Today, garlic remains a champion of gut health and is known for balancing harmful and beneficial bacteria.

Active Compounds and Their Benefits

Garlic contains allicin, a sulfur-rich compound responsible for many of its health benefits. When garlic is crushed, allicin is released, providing antibacterial, antifungal, and antiviral properties. These actions help balance the gut microbiome, promoting the growth of beneficial bacteria while fighting off harmful pathogens like *Helicobacter pylori* and *Candida*. Garlic is also rich in prebiotics, compounds that nourish beneficial gut bacteria, helping them thrive and maintain harmony in the digestive tract.

Most Potent Method of Ingestion

Raw garlic, finely chopped or crushed, provides the most potent dose of allicin and other beneficial compounds. For those who find raw garlic too strong, garlic-infused oils or capsules can be used for more gentle but still effective gut support. A garlic poultice, applied to the abdomen, can also help soothe digestive discomfort while providing systemic antibacterial benefits.

Simple Recipe: Garlic-Infused Olive Oil

Crush 3–4 garlic cloves and allow them to sit for 10 minutes. Heat half a cup of olive oil gently and add the garlic, letting it infuse over low heat for 15–20 minutes. Strain and store in a glass bottle. Take a teaspoon with meals to support gut health or use in cooking.

Best Herbs to Use Together

Garlic pairs excellently with ginger, another powerful gut balancer, and turmeric, which helps reduce inflammation in the digestive tract. Combining garlic with fennel or caraway can enhance its digestive effects, particularly when used to prevent bloating and gas.

10. Berberine (*Berberis vulgaris*)

Historical Context

Harvested from the roots and bark of the barberry plant, berberine has a rich history in traditional Chinese and Ayurvedic medicine. It has been used for centuries to treat digestive disorders, bacterial infections, and inflammatory conditions. Its golden hue, often referred to as "the golden thread," signifies its powerful ability to restore balance in the body, particularly within the gut. In the modern world, berberine has gained renewed attention as a natural remedy for digestive health, regulating gut flora and combating harmful microorganisms.

Active Compounds and Their Benefits

Berberine is an alkaloid, known for its potent antimicrobial, anti-inflammatory, and antifungal properties. It helps balance gut flora by selectively inhibiting harmful bacteria, including *Escherichia coli* and *Clostridium difficile*, while promoting the growth of beneficial bacteria like *Lactobacillus* and *Bifidobacterium*. Berberine also has anti-inflammatory effects on the gut lining, helping soothe irritation and inflammation, which are often at the root of digestive discomfort. This potent compound also helps regulate blood sugar levels, making it a valuable ally for overall metabolic and gut health.

Most Potent Method of Ingestion

Tinctures and capsules are the most effective ways to consume berberine for gut health, offering a concentrated dose that can swiftly target imbalances. A tincture, in particular, is easily absorbed by the body, ensuring maximum benefit. Powdered berberine can also be encapsulated for ease of use or added to smoothies for a convenient daily boost.

Simple Recipe: Berberine Tincture

Place 1 tablespoon of powdered berberine root in a glass jar and cover it with 4 ounces of alcohol (vodka or brandy). Seal tightly and store in a cool, dark place for 4–6 weeks, shaking occasionally. Strain and store in a dark glass bottle. Take 1–2 droppers full daily to promote gut health and balance gut flora.

Best Herbs to Use Together

Berberine works well with goldenseal and Oregon grape root, which both contain complementary alkaloids that enhance its antimicrobial effects. Combine with milk thistle for added liver support, because the liver plays a crucial role in detoxification and gut health. Together, these herbs form a powerful team to restore balance to the digestive system.

SUPPORTING LIVER FUNCTION

11. Milk Thistle (*Silybum marianum*)

Historical Context

Milk thistle has long been revered as a liver protector with its delicate purple blooms and spiky leaves. Its medicinal use dates back over 2,000 years to ancient Greece and Rome, where it was prescribed for a range of ailments, particularly those affecting the liver and gallbladder. Known as the "liver's knight in shining armor," milk thistle was celebrated in medieval European herbal medicine for its detoxifying effects. Today, it remains one of the most trusted herbs in modern herbalism for liver support and healing.

Active Compounds and Their Benefits

The secret behind milk thistle's liver-healing power lies in silymarin, a potent complex of flavonoids found primarily in the seeds. Silymarin is renowned for its antioxidant, anti-inflammatory, and hepatoprotective properties. It not only helps repair liver cells damaged by toxins, alcohol, and disease but also strengthens the liver's outer membrane, which makes it harder for harmful substances to enter. Milk thistle also stimulates bile production, improving digestion and supporting the liver's natural detoxification processes.

Most Potent Method of Ingestion

Milk thistle is most effective when taken as a tincture or capsule, because these methods deliver a concentrated dose of silymarin directly to the liver. For a gentler, more soothing approach, a milk thistle infusion (tea) can be used. However, due to their potency and quick absorption, tinctures are the preferred method for liver detoxification and regeneration.

Simple Recipe: Milk Thistle Tincture

Place 1 tablespoon of crushed seeds in a glass jar and cover with 4 ounces of alcohol (vodka or brandy). Seal the jar tightly and store it in a cool, dark place for 4–6 weeks, shaking occasionally. Strain the tincture into a dark glass bottle. Take 20–30 drops daily to support liver health and detoxification.

Best Herbs to Use Together

Milk thistle pairs beautifully with dandelion root, another liver-supporting herb, for enhanced detoxification. Combining it with turmeric boosts its anti-inflammatory effects, while burdock root enhances milk thistle's ability to cleanse the blood and promote overall liver function.

12. Schisandra (*Schisandra chinensis*)

Historical Context

Known as the "five-flavor berry" in traditional Chinese medicine, Schisandra has been cherished for thousands of years as a tonic for vitality. Ancient Chinese emperors and royalty consumed Schisandra to promote longevity, enhance mental clarity, and strengthen the body's resistance to stress. In Taoist practices, Schisandra was regarded as one of the most powerful adaptogens, helping the body adapt to both physical and emotional challenges. Today, its use in herbalism continues, especially for supporting liver function and protecting against environmental toxins.

Active Compounds and Their Benefits

Schisandra's power lies in its lignans, unique compounds that offer hepatoprotective effects. Lignans help the liver regenerate cells and enhance its detoxification processes, making it more efficient at removing harmful substances from the body. Schisandra also increases glutathione production, the liver's most powerful antioxidant, which helps neutralize free radicals and reduce oxidative stress. Additionally, Schisandra supports bile flow, promoting digestion and helping the liver process fats more effectively.

Most Potent Method of Ingestion

Schisandra is most potent when taken as a tincture or powder. Its adaptogenic properties shine when consumed regularly, allowing it to gently nourish the liver over time. Capsules and powders made from Schisandra berries can also be effective, although tinctures are ideal for those seeking a concentrated form of liver support.

Simple Recipe: Schisandra Tincture

Combine half a cup of dried berries and 8 ounces of alcohol (vodka or brandy) in a glass jar. Seal the jar and store it in a dark place for 4–6 weeks, shaking occasionally. Strain and bottle in a dark container. Take 1–2 droppers daily to support liver function and protect against toxins.

Best Herbs to Use Together

Schisandra pairs wonderfully with milk thistle, amplifying its liver-protecting effects. It also combines well with turmeric for reducing inflammation, and with burdock root to enhance detoxification. Together, these herbs form a powerful team to restore balance and strength to the liver.

CONSTIPATION RELIEF

13. Cascara Sagrada (*Rhamnus purshiana*)

Historical Context

Cascara Sagrada, or "sacred bark," has been used for centuries by Indigenous peoples of the Pacific Northwest for its gentle yet effective laxative properties. Traditionally used by Native American tribes, this bark was a remedy for digestive issues and a symbol of holistic healing. With its history steeped in nature's wisdom, cascara sagrada is often regarded as a natural remedy for those seeking to restore harmony to their digestive systems. Its role in herbal medicine gained prominence in the late 19th century, and today, it remains a trusted ally in alleviating constipation.

Active Compounds and Their Benefits

The healing power of cascara sagrada lies within its anthraquinone compounds, which stimulate peristalsis—the rhythmic contractions of the intestines. These compounds not only encourage bowel movements but also help to soften stool, making it easier to pass. In addition, cascara sagrada contains tannins that possess astringent properties, which can aid in toning the intestinal walls and improving digestive function. Its gentle nature makes it an ideal option for those seeking relief from constipation without the harsh effects often associated with synthetic laxatives.

Most Potent Method of Ingestion

Cascara sagrada is most potent when taken as a tincture or dried bark infusion. The tincture allows for quick absorption, making it effective for those in need of immediate relief. When brewed as a tea, it provides a soothing experience while still promoting healthy bowel function. It's essential to start with a small dose to assess individual tolerance.

Simple Recipe: Cascara Sagrada Tea

Steep 1 teaspoon of dried bark in hot water for 10–15 minutes. Strain and enjoy the soothing brew to promote regular bowel movements. It's advisable to drink this tea no more than once a day.

Best Herbs to Use Together

Cascara sagrada pairs well with ginger, which helps to calm the digestive system while promoting healthy gut motility. Combining it with fennel can enhance its effects, because fennel aids digestion and reduces bloating, making for a well-rounded approach to digestive health.

14. Flaxseed (*Linum usitatissimum*)

Historical Context

Flaxseed, often referred to as "the golden seed," has a rich history that spans thousands of years. Ancient Egyptians valued flaxseed for its health benefits, incorporating it into their diets and using its oil for skin treatments. In medieval Europe, it was cultivated for its nutritional properties and its fibers, which were used to make linen. Today, flaxseed has emerged as a superfood, celebrated for its high omega-3 fatty acid content and fiber-rich profile. It is a staple in the quest for digestive health and overall well-being.

Active Compounds and Their Benefits

Flaxseed is a soluble and insoluble fiber powerhouse that plays a crucial role in maintaining regular bowel movements. The soluble fiber absorbs water and forms a gel-like consistency, softening stool and facilitating its passage through the intestines. Meanwhile, insoluble fiber adds bulk to the stool, promoting healthy elimination. Additionally, flaxseed contains lignans—phytoestrogens that provide antioxidant benefits and support hormonal balance. Its anti-inflammatory properties further contribute to gut health, creating a favorable environment for digestive processes.

Most Potent Method of Ingestion

Flaxseed is most effective when ground, because this enhances its bioavailability and allows the body to absorb its nutrients more easily. Ground flaxseed can be added to smoothies, yogurt, or oatmeal for a nutritious boost. Whole flaxseeds can also be soaked in water to create a gel-like consistency that aids digestion and serves as a natural laxative.

Simple Recipe: Flaxseed Gel

Combine 2 tablespoons of ground flaxseed and 1 cup of water in a saucepan. Bring to a boil, then reduce heat and simmer for 10–15 minutes, stirring frequently. Once it reaches a gel-like consistency, strain it through a fine mesh sieve. Allow to cool and store in the refrigerator for up to a week. Take 1–2 tablespoons daily to support digestive health and relieve constipation.

Best Herbs to Use Together

Flaxseed works harmoniously with chia seeds, because both are rich in fiber and promote gut health. Additionally, combining flaxseed with cascara sagrada can create a powerful duo for combating constipation while maintaining digestive balance.

DIARRHEA MANAGEMENT

15. Blackberry Leaf (*Rubus fruticosus*)

Historical Context

Blackberry leaf has been cherished throughout history as a potent ally in natural healing. Traditionally used by herbalists and Indigenous peoples, this humble leaf has found its place in folk medicine across Europe, Asia, and the Americas. Ancient Romans recognized its value for both culinary and medicinal purposes, utilizing it to soothe various ailments. Today, blackberry leaf remains a staple in herbal remedies, revered for its delicious fruit and health-boosting properties, particularly in managing digestive disturbances.

Active Compounds and Their Benefits

Rich in tannins, blackberry leaf acts as a natural astringent, helping to tighten and tone the intestinal lining. This property makes it particularly effective in reducing diarrhea, because it helps to slow down bowel movements and restore balance to the digestive system. Additionally, blackberry leaf is packed with vitamins C and K, along with antioxidants that support overall health. Its anti-inflammatory properties also contribute to soothing irritated digestive tissues, making it a gentle yet effective remedy for those experiencing diarrhea.

Most Potent Method of Ingestion

Blackberry leaf is most potent when consumed as a tea or infusion. The brewing process extracts its beneficial compounds, making them readily available for the body to absorb. This method not only offers digestive support but also provides a comforting and aromatic experience.

Simple Recipe: Blackberry Leaf Tea

Steep 1 tablespoon of dried blackberry leaf in 1 cup of hot water for 10–15 minutes. Strain and enjoy this soothing tea to help alleviate diarrhea symptoms and support digestive health.

Best Herbs to Use Together

Blackberry leaf pairs well with chamomile, which calms the digestive system and adds an additional layer of soothing properties. Combining it with peppermint can enhance its effectiveness, because peppermint aids digestion and provides a refreshing flavor profile.

16. White Oak Bark (*Quercus alba*)

Historical Context

White oak bark has been utilized for centuries in traditional herbal medicine. Native American tribes and early settlers used it for its astringent properties. Historically, it was used to treat various ailments, from digestive disorders to skin conditions. The bark of the white oak tree is valued for its medicinal qualities and sturdy wood, symbolizing strength and resilience. Today, this timeless herb continues to be a trusted remedy for those seeking relief from diarrhea and other digestive disturbances.

Active Compounds and Their Benefits

The powerful astringent properties of white oak bark come from its high tannin content, which helps to constrict tissues and reduce inflammation in the intestines. This makes it an effective remedy for diarrhea because it helps to tighten the bowel lining and slow down excessive fluid loss. Additionally, white oak bark is rich in antioxidants, promoting overall health and supporting the body in combating oxidative stress. Its anti-inflammatory effects can also soothe the gastrointestinal tract, offering comfort during digestive upsets.

Most Potent Method of Ingestion

White oak bark is best taken as a decoction or herbal infusion. Boiling the bark extracts its beneficial tannins and other compounds, enhancing its effectiveness in treating diarrhea while also providing a warming and comforting drink.

Simple Recipe: White Oak Bark Decoction

Bring 1 cup of water to a boil and add 1 teaspoon of dried white oak bark. Simmer for 15–20 minutes, then strain. Enjoy this potent decoction to help manage diarrhea and support digestive health.

Best Herbs to Use Together

White oak bark pairs well with peppermint for a soothing effect, because peppermint can calm the digestive system and enhance the overall flavor of the decoction. Additionally, combining it with ginger can provide anti-inflammatory benefits and further ease digestive discomfort.

REDUCING ACID REFLUX

17. Mastic Gum (*Pistacia lentiscus*)

Historical Context

Harvested from the resin of the mastic tree on the Greek island of Chios, mastic gum has been treasured for thousands of years. Known as "the tears of Chios," this fragrant resin was once worth its weight in gold, prized by ancient civilizations like the Greeks, Romans, and Egyptians for its medicinal properties. Mastic gum was traditionally used for a variety of ailments, including digestive issues and mouth ulcers. Revered in ancient healing texts and Mediterranean cultures, it continues to be cherished for its ability to soothe and protect the digestive system, particularly in reducing acid reflux.

Active Compounds and Their Benefits

Mastic gum contains powerful compounds, including masticadienonic acid and masticadienolic acid, known for their anti-inflammatory and antibacterial properties. These compounds help protect the stomach lining from the corrosive effects of stomach acid, making it especially effective in reducing acid reflux and soothing irritation. Mastic gum's ability to reduce *Helicobacter pylori* bacteria, a common culprit in gastric issues, adds to its healing repertoire. Its gentle yet potent action on the digestive system promotes healing and repair while reducing discomfort caused by excess acid.

Most Potent Method of Ingestion

Mastic gum is best consumed as a capsule supplement or chewable resin. Chewing mastic gum stimulates saliva production, which helps neutralize stomach acid and promote healing of the digestive tract. For those who prefer a more concentrated dose, tinctures or capsules offer an efficient and powerful way to harness its benefits.

Simple Recipe: Mastic Gum Capsules

Take one or two capsules with water, preferably before meals, to help soothe acid reflux and protect the stomach lining.

Best Herbs to Use Together

Mastic gum works synergistically with licorice root, which also soothes and protects the stomach lining. Pairing it with marshmallow root adds another layer of soothing mucilage to calm irritated tissues. Together, these herbs create a potent blend for reducing acid reflux and promoting digestive health.

18. Papaya Leaf (*Carica papaya*)

Historical Context

Papaya has long been a sacred fruit in tropical regions, particularly in the Caribbean and Central America, where it was referred to as the "fruit of the angels" by Christopher Columbus. While the fruit is well known for its delicious taste, the leaves have a history of medicinal use that spans centuries. Traditional healers in South America and Southeast Asia have used papaya leaf for digestive disorders, recognizing its ability to aid digestion and reduce discomfort. Today, papaya leaf is celebrated for its role in relieving acid reflux and improving overall digestive health.

Active Compounds and Their Benefits

Papaya leaf contains an abundance of digestive enzymes, particularly papain and chymopapain, which aid in breaking down proteins and enhancing digestion. These enzymes help reduce acid reflux by improving digestion and preventing the buildup of excess stomach acid. The leaf also contains anti-inflammatory and antioxidant compounds such as flavonoids and tannins, which soothe the digestive tract and promote the healing of irritated tissues. Its ability to balance acid levels and support proper digestion makes papaya leaf a valuable ally in reducing acid reflux.

Most Potent Method of Ingestion

Papaya leaf tea or tincture is the most effective method of ingestion for addressing acid reflux. The gentle heat of the tea or concentrated form of a tincture allows the digestive enzymes to be easily absorbed, aiding in digestion and soothing discomfort.

Simple Recipe: Papaya Leaf Tea

Steep 1 teaspoon of dried papaya leaf in 1 cup of hot water for 10 minutes. Strain and enjoy this soothing tea to reduce acid reflux and support digestion.

Best Herbs to Use Together

Papaya leaf pairs well with ginger, which further supports digestion and helps neutralize stomach acid. Combining it with fennel can relieve acid reflux by calming the digestive system and preventing bloating. Together, these herbs offer a comprehensive approach to reducing acid reflux and promoting healthy digestion.

APPETITE STIMULATION

19. Wormwood (*Artemisia absinthium*)

Historical Context

Wormwood, a plant steeped in both mystery and legend, has been used since ancient times for its powerful medicinal properties. The Greeks and Romans cherished it as a remedy for digestive complaints and to stimulate the appetite. It gained fame in European herbal traditions for its role in crafting absinthe, a potent and once-forbidden elixir. Although its reputation as a hallucinogenic has shadowed its therapeutic potential, herbalists still turn to wormwood for its bitter, appetite-stimulating qualities.

Active Compounds and Their Benefits

Wormwood's secret lies in its intense bitter compounds, particularly absinthin and anabsinthin, which are responsible for stimulating the digestive system. These compounds increase the production of digestive juices, bile, and stomach acid, making the body ready to digest food efficiently. Wormwood effectively wakes the body's hunger signals by promoting the secretion of saliva, gastric acids, and enzymes, making it a reliable herb for those suffering from poor appetite or sluggish digestion. Wormwood also has antimicrobial properties, adding to its therapeutic versatility.

Most Potent Method of Ingestion

Wormwood tincture is the most potent and effective way to stimulate appetite. The bitter taste, although strong, triggers the digestive response almost immediately, making it ideal when consumed 15–30 minutes before meals. Alternatively, a small infusion can also offer digestive support, but tinctures allow for more precise dosing and quicker effects.

Simple Recipe: Wormwood Tincture

Steep 1 teaspoon of dried wormwood in 1 cup of alcohol (vodka or brandy) for at least 2 weeks, shaking the jar daily. Strain the tincture and store in a dark bottle. Take 10–15 drops in water 15 minutes before meals to stimulate appetite.

Best Herbs to Use Together

Wormwood pairs beautifully with ginger to enhance digestive secretions and improve circulation. It also complements gentian root, another powerful bitter herb, to further stimulate appetite and improve overall digestive health. Together, these herbs create a potent blend for those needing digestive support and appetite stimulation.

20. Angelica (Angelica archangelica)

Historical Context

Angelica, with its towering stalks and fragrant roots, has long been a symbol of protection and healing. In medieval times, it was believed to ward off evil spirits and plagues, and its very name, *archangelica*, reflects its association with divine protection. Historically, angelica was used in both European and Chinese medicine to treat digestive ailments and to stimulate the appetite. Revered for its warming, aromatic properties, angelica remains a powerful herb for enhancing digestion and awakening the body's natural hunger.

Active Compounds and Their Benefits

Angelica's key active compounds include volatile oils such as α-pinene and limonene, which stimulate digestive secretions and enhance appetite. Coumarins, flavonoids, and bitter principles in the root work synergistically to soothe digestive discomfort and stimulate bile flow. Angelica is particularly effective for those who have lost their appetite due to illness or stress, because its warming nature gently encourages the body to produce digestive enzymes, increasing hunger while improving nutrient absorption.

Most Potent Method of Ingestion

Angelica root tea is the most effective way to stimulate appetite and support digestive function. The heat of the infusion helps release its aromatic oils and bitter compounds, making it easy for the body to absorb. A tincture is also highly effective, offering a more concentrated dose of its active constituents. Both preparations are best consumed before meals to awaken the appetite.

Simple Recipe: Angelica Root Tea

Steep 1 teaspoon of dried angelica root in 1 cup of boiling water for 10–15 minutes. Strain and drink 20 minutes before meals to stimulate appetite and improve digestion.

Best Herbs to Use Together

Angelica pairs well with fennel to support digestion and alleviate bloating. Combined with dandelion root, it enhances bile production and promotes a more efficient digestive process. Together, these herbs create a well-rounded formula for encouraging appetite and maintaining a healthy digestive system.

HERBS FOR
RESPIRATORY CONDITIONS

CLEARING MUCUS AND CONGESTION

21. Mullein (*Verbascum thapsus*)

Historical Context

Mullein, often called the "lung herb," has existed in herbal traditions across Europe and North America for centuries. Known for its towering yellow-flowered stalks, this hardy plant was revered by the ancient Greeks and Romans for its gentle yet powerful effects on respiratory health. Native American tribes used mullein leaves to remedy lung-related ailments, from colds to chronic coughs, creating smoke infusions and teas that would gently ease the breath.

Active Compounds and Their Benefits

Mullein contains mucilage, saponins, and flavonoids, which work harmoniously to soothe the respiratory tract. Mucilage provides a protective coating effect that reduces inflammation in the throat and lungs, while saponins act as mild expectorants to help break down and expel mucus. Flavonoids enhance mullein's natural anti-inflammatory and antiviral qualities, further supporting respiratory health.

Most Potent Method of Ingestion

Mullein's leaves and flowers are best enjoyed as a tea or tincture to promote clear breathing. Its mucilaginous properties fully emerge in tea form, coating the throat and loosening mucus. Although more concentrated, the tincture preserves the herb's expectorant effects in a convenient format.

Simple Recipe: Mullein Leaf Tea

Steep 1–2 teaspoons of dried leaves in 1 cup of boiling water for 10 minutes, strain carefully to remove fine hairs, and sip slowly. Enjoy to soothe the lungs and clear mucus.

Best Herbs to Use Together

Mullein pairs beautifully with marshmallow root for a soothing blend of elecampane, which enhances expectorant properties, creating a holistic remedy for respiratory congestion and irritation.

22. Elecampane (*Inula helenium*)

Historical Context

Elecampane, with its bright yellow petals and rich herbal aroma, was cherished by the ancient Greeks and Romans and even used by Pliny the Elder as a tonic for the lungs. The name *Inula helenium* draws from the myth of Helen of Troy, who was believed to have carried elecampane roots with her. This herb was once a common remedy for coughs and respiratory issues and a powerful ally for lung health in European folk medicine.

Active Compounds and Their Benefits

Elecampane is rich in inulin, a polysaccharide that soothes irritated respiratory tissue and acts as a prebiotic for gut health. Alantolactone, a key compound, functions as a natural decongestant and expectorant, while sesquiterpene lactones contribute to its antimicrobial effects, making elecampane a powerful choice for respiratory infections.

Most Potent Method of Ingestion

A decoction made from the root is the most potent way to harness elecampane's lung-clearing benefits. The extended simmering extracts the inulin and alantolactone compounds effectively, promoting respiratory clearance and soothing inflamed passages.

Simple Recipe: Elecampane Root Decoction

Simmer 1 tablespoon of the root in 1 cups of water over low heat for 20–30 minutes, strain, and sip warm to relieve congestion and support lung function.

Best Herbs to Use Together

Pair elecampane with mullein for a powerful decongestant blend or ginger to boost its warming properties, creating an effective remedy for stubborn mucus and congestion.

SOOTHING COUGHS

23. Marshmallow Root (*Althaea officinalis*)

Historical Context

Marshmallow root has been a cherished remedy since antiquity, calming the throats and spirits of many. The Egyptians are said to have combined it with honey for both confection and medicine, while the Greeks and Romans used it as a treatment for sore throats and respiratory ailments. Its namesake confectionery, "marshmallow," originated from the sap of this gentle plant, celebrated for its ability to soothe discomfort with a silken touch.

Active Compounds and Their Benefits

Rich in mucilage, marshmallow root acts as a balm, coating the throat and relieving inflammation. This thick gel-like mucilage calms irritation along mucosal surfaces, easing the urge to cough. Flavonoids in the root are anti-inflammatory, reducing redness and swelling, while polysaccharides offer immune support. This makes marshmallows a restorative choice for irritated throats. These components work in unison to create a shield over raw tissue, inviting healing and peace.

Most Potent Method of Ingestion

Marshmallow root shines best as a cold infusion, where its mucilage fully unfurls, creating a soothing, viscous liquid that coats the throat. Steeping marshmallow root in cool water over time allows the mucilage to develop without losing potency, resulting in a drink as comforting as it is gentle.

Simple Recipe: Marshmallow Root Cold Infusion

Combine 1 tablespoon of marshmallow root and 1 cup of cold water in a glass jar, cover, and let it infuse overnight or for at least 4 hours. Strain and sip slowly to calm throat irritation and ease coughs.

Best Herbs to Use Together

Marshmallow root pairs wonderfully with slippery elm bark for extra soothing properties or wild cherry bark to calm the cough reflex. Together, they form a nurturing blend that offers tender relief to the respiratory system.

24. Wild Cherry Bark (*Prunus serotina*)

Historical Context

Wild cherry bark, treasured for its velvety power to still the cough, has long been used in Native American and European herbal traditions. Indigenous tribes would chew the bark to relieve coughs and colds, while settlers crafted it into syrups to soothe persistent coughs and irritation. This bark, a symbol of nature's quiet strength, harnesses the power to hush the lungs' unease.

Active Compounds and Their Benefits

The power of wild cherry bark lies in its naturally occurring cyanogenic glycosides, which convert into small amounts of hydrocyanic acid, relaxing and calming the cough reflex. Tannins offer astringent qualities, reducing inflammation and drying up excess mucus in the throat. The bark also holds flavonoids, which provide antioxidant support and help to reduce throat irritation. Altogether, these compounds create an antitussive remedy, encouraging stillness and relief.

Most Potent Method of Ingestion

Wild cherry bark is at its most effective as a syrup. The gentle heat of the preparation process draws out the bark's active compounds, creating a liquid remedy that coats and comforts the throat, softens coughs, and offers lasting relief.

Simple Recipe: Wild Cherry Bark Syrup

Simmer 1 tablespoon of the bark in 1 cup of water over low heat for 20 minutes, strain, and let cool slightly before adding 1 cup of honey. Take 1–2 teaspoons as needed for cough relief.

Best Herbs to Use Together

Wild cherry bark blends beautifully with marshmallow root or slippery elm to enhance its soothing effect, creating a gentle, potent syrup to quiet coughs and promote calm.

REDUCING INFLAMMATION IN THE AIRWAYS

25. Turmeric (*Curcuma longa*)

Historical Context

The golden root turmeric has woven its vibrant hue into the healing and culinary arts. Originating in South Asia, this "spice of life" has been used in Ayurveda for over 4,000 years to treat a spectrum of ailments, from wounds to respiratory conditions. It's radiant color and earthy aroma carry the wisdom of ancient medicine, blending warmth with potent healing power.

Active Compounds and Their Benefits

Curcumin, turmeric's primary active compound, is a remarkable anti-inflammatory agent that works by inhibiting inflammatory pathways in the body. This polyphenol's antioxidant properties support respiratory health by reducing oxidative stress and inflammation in the airways. Turmeric also contains volatile oils and sesquiterpenes, which contribute to its anti-inflammatory and antimicrobial effects and help to defend against environmental irritants. Together, these compounds create a formidable force against respiratory inflammation, easing discomfort, and promoting clear, calm breathing.

Most Potent Method of Ingestion

Turmeric is most effective as a warm, golden milk infusion. This gentle remedy offers lasting relief for inflamed airways when combined with a pinch of black pepper, which enhances curcumin absorption. The warmth of the drink soothes irritation, while turmeric's curative properties reduce inflammation from within.

Simple Recipe: Turmeric Golden Milk

Instructions: Heat 1 cup of milk in a small saucepan, then whisk in 1 teaspoon of turmeric and a pinch of black pepper. Simmer gently for a few minutes, then sweeten with honey if desired. Drink warm for soothing relief.

Best Herbs to Use Together

Turmeric pairs well with ginger for added anti-inflammatory benefits or Boswellia for a deeper reduction of respiratory inflammation. Together, these herbs form a powerful blend to support calm and clear breathing.

26. Boswellia (*Boswellia serrata*)

Historical Context

Boswellia, or frankincense tree, has been used in Ayurvedic and Middle Eastern traditions for thousands of years. Its resin, known as "tears of the tree," was used in ancient rituals and medicine, symbolizing purification and healing. The gum resin derived from Boswellia has long been valued for treating inflammatory conditions, making it a revered remedy for respiratory issues and overall wellness.

Active Compounds and Their Benefits

Boswellia is rich in boswellic acids, which are powerful anti-inflammatory agents that inhibit leukotrienes, molecules responsible for inflammation in the respiratory tract. These acids reduce swelling, helping to ease breathing in inflamed airways. Boswellia's additional anti-arthritic and immune-boosting properties further aid the respiratory system by calming inflammation and promoting overall resilience against irritants and pathogens.

Most Potent Method of Ingestion

Boswellia works best as a tincture, where the concentrated extract delivers boswellic acids directly into the body, reducing inflammation quickly and effectively. If taken daily, Boswellia tincture can support respiratory health by easing inflammation and allowing airways to open more fully.

Simple Recipe: Boswellia Tincture

Place 1 teaspoon of Boswellia resin in a glass jar, cover with 1 cup of vodka, and seal. Let sit for 4–6 weeks, shaking occasionally. Strain and store in a dark glass bottle. Take 1–2 droppers daily for respiratory support.

Best Herbs to Use Together

Boswellia harmonizes well with turmeric for enhanced anti-inflammatory effects, as well as licorice root, to soothe and protect the respiratory tract. Together, they create a holistic approach to reducing airway inflammation and fostering lung health.

IMMUNE SUPPORT FOR RESPIRATORY HEALTH

27. Astragalus (*Astragalus membranaceus*)

Historical Context

Astragalus has been used in traditional Chinese medicine for over 2,000 years. It was known as "Huang Qi" or "yellow leader," symbolizing strength and longevity. In ancient China, this herb was revered as a potent immune tonic, used to fortify the body's defenses and promote vitality. Today, astragalus remains a celebrated herb for its capacity to bolster immune resilience, especially in respiratory health, helping the body to resist seasonal ailments and environmental stressors.

Active Compounds and Their Benefits

Astragalus contains polysaccharides and flavonoids, known to stimulate immune activity and strengthen cellular defenses. These compounds enhance the activity of macrophages, the body's frontline defenders, while also supporting lung and respiratory function by boosting white blood cell counts. Astragalus is rich in saponins and antioxidants, which help combat oxidative stress, reducing the likelihood of respiratory infections and inflammation.

Most Potent Method of Ingestion

For immune support, the astragalus root shines when prepared as a gentle decoction. Slow simmering extracts its immune-boosting polysaccharides. A daily cup can serve as a protective shield, particularly when respiratory health is vulnerable.

Simple Recipe: Astragalus Immune Decoction

Add 1–2 tablespoons of astragalus root to 4 cups of water in a pot. Bring to a boil, then reduce to a simmer for 30–45 minutes. Strain and sip throughout the day.

Best Herbs to Use Together

Astragalus beautifully combines with reishi mushroom for amplified immune support and elderberry for additional respiratory defense. Together, these herbs create a powerful immune tonic that guards against infections and strengthens respiratory resilience.

28. Reishi Mushroom (*Ganoderma lucidum*)

Historical Context

Reishi, known as the "mushroom of immortality," has been a staple in East Asian medicine for thousands of years. Traditionally reserved for emperors and elite healers, this sacred fungus was believed to bestow longevity and fortify both body and spirit. Reishi's adaptogenic nature makes it ideal for modern respiratory health, aiding in stress management and immune resilience—two crucial elements for overall respiratory wellness.

Active Compounds and Their Benefits

Reishi is packed with beta-glucans, polysaccharides that modulate immune function, helping the body adapt to stress and combat infections. Triterpenoids within reishi exhibit anti-inflammatory and antioxidant properties, supporting lung health by reducing oxidative damage and inflammatory responses. As an adaptogen, reishi uniquely enhances the body's resilience against respiratory ailments.

Most Potent Method of Ingestion

Reishi is most potent for hot water extraction, such as tea or decoction, which allows the polysaccharides and triterpenes to infuse into the water. This preparation helps amplify the mushroom's immune-boosting effect, creating a rich, earthy tea that gently supports immunity and respiratory function.

Simple Recipe: Reishi Immune Tea

Place 1–2 reishi slices (or 1 teaspoon of dried reishi powder) in a pot with 4 cups of water, bring to a boil, then simmer for 30–60 minutes. Strain and enjoy a warm immune tonic.

Best Herbs to Use Together

Reishi pairs well with astragalus to strengthen immune defenses, as well as Schisandra for added adaptogen support and resilience. Together, these herbs form a potent immune shield, promoting respiratory health and helping the body withstand seasonal stressors.

HERBS FOR RESPIRATORY CONDITIONS

ANTIMICROBIAL, ANTI-INFLAMMATORY, IMMUNE SUPPORT

29. Goldenseal (*Hydrastis canadensis*)

Historical Context

Goldenseal was cherished by Indigenous North American tribes such as the Cherokee, who relied on its vibrant yellow root for medicinal and ceremonial purposes. Known as the "golden healer," goldenseal's antibacterial and healing powers have been used for centuries, particularly in treating infections of the respiratory and digestive tracts. Traditionally, the root was chewed or infused in water to create a protective tonic, making it a staple in traditional practices for respiratory health.

Active Compounds and Benefits

The defining quality of goldenseal lies in its berberine content, an alkaloid that boasts remarkable antimicrobial, anti-inflammatory, and immune-supportive properties. Berberine's action inhibits the growth of bacteria, fungi, and other pathogens, making it highly effective against respiratory infections such as bronchitis or sinusitis. Studies show that berberine also reduces inflammation, which can calm irritated respiratory tissues while supporting faster recovery.

Most Potent Method of Ingestion

Goldenseal tinctures or extracts maximize the impact of berberine, because the compounds are quickly absorbed into the bloodstream. Small, measured doses of tincture provide immediate support in acute conditions, working to clear bacterial strains while maintaining a balanced immune response. Regular use of the tincture in low doses can also act as a preventative measure during peak respiratory infection seasons.

Simple Recipe: Goldenseal Antimicrobial Tincture

Combine 1 part dried goldenseal root with 5 parts vodka or brandy in a glass jar. Shake well and seal tightly, storing the jar in a cool, dark place for 2 weeks. Shake it daily. After 2 weeks, strain and store the liquid in a dark bottle. When respiratory infections arise, take 15–20 drops in warm water up to three times daily.

Best Herbs to Use Together

To enhance respiratory protection, blend goldenseal with echinacea or add to a thyme steam inhalation to clear nasal passages.

30. Oregano (*Origanum vulgare*)

Historical Context

Oregano, with a name meaning "joy of the mountains," has been popular since ancient Greece for its healing abilities. It was commonly burned as incense or crushed into healing salves to ward off infection and cleanse living spaces. Its strong, savory aroma reflects its potency, and across Mediterranean folk medicine, it has been used in teas, oils, and poultices to protect against various ailments, especially respiratory infections.

Active Compounds and Benefits

Carvacrol and thymol are the primary active compounds in oregano, each with significant antimicrobial and antifungal properties. These compounds disrupt the membranes of bacteria and other pathogens, helping to clear respiratory infections and support respiratory health. Carvacrol, in particular, has shown effectiveness in breaking down bacterial biofilms, providing robust respiratory support against common ailments like colds, sinus infections, and coughs.

Most Potent Method of Ingestion

Oregano oil delivers its benefits in highly concentrated form, offering a powerful antimicrobial effect when taken in capsules or diluted in a carrier oil for steam inhalation. Its ability to eliminate bacteria and fungi makes it ideal for respiratory care, providing targeted relief while fighting pathogens in the lungs and sinuses.

Simple Recipe: Oregano Steam Inhalation

Add 2–3 drops of oregano oil to a bowl of steaming water. Drape a towel over your head and lean over the bowl, inhaling deeply for five minutes. The warm vapor helps carry the oregano's essential oils into the respiratory system, clearing sinus congestion and reducing bacterial buildup.

Best Herbs to Use Together

Pair with thyme or eucalyptus for an enhanced steam treatment, or mix with ginger to create a warming tonic that boosts immunity and wards off respiratory infections.

HERBS FOR RESPIRATORY CONDITIONS
OPENING THE AIRWAYS

31. Lobelia (*Lobelia inflata*)

Historical Context

Celebrated by Native American tribes, lobelia has long been recognized for its bronchodilating properties, earning the nickname "Indian tobacco." Since it is used in traditional medicine to treat various respiratory conditions, lobelia has found its place in herbal practice as a remedy to support ease of breath. Herbalists have utilized this plant for centuries, steeping its leaves and flowers into infusions and tinctures, allowing its potent effects to flow through the body like a gentle breeze.

Active Compounds and Benefits

The active alkaloids in lobelia, particularly lobeline, function as a natural bronchodilator, relaxing and widening the airways. This makes it an invaluable ally for those struggling with asthma or chronic bronchitis, as it can help alleviate wheezing and tightness in the chest. Lobelia's unique action not only eases respiratory distress but also promotes overall lung health by encouraging deeper, more effective breathing.

Most Potent Method of Ingestion

Lobelia is most effective when taken as a tincture or in an infusion. The tincture form allows for rapid absorption, making it ideal for acute respiratory situations. A few drops in warm water can provide immediate relief, opening the airways and encouraging smoother airflow. Care should be taken with dosages because3 lobelia can be potent; thus, consulting a qualified herbalist is recommended.

Simple Recipe: Lobelia and Mullein Infusion

Combine 1 teaspoon of dried lobelia leaves with 1 teaspoon of dried mullein in a cup of boiling water. Steep for 10 minutes, strain, and sip slowly to ease tightness in the chest and promote easier breathing.

Best Herbs to Use Together

Lobelia can be paired with peppermint or eucalyptus for enhanced respiratory support. This amplifies its bronchodilating effects and creates a soothing synergy that helps clear the airways.

32. Grindelia (*Grindelia robusta*)

Historical Context

Traditionally embraced by Indigenous peoples of North America, grindelia has been cherished for its ability to alleviate respiratory distress and promote clear breathing. Known as gum plant for its sticky, resinous leaves, this robust herb has played a vital role in folk medicine, often prepared as infusions or syrups to soothe the lungs and ease respiratory discomfort.

Active Compounds and Benefits

Grindelia contains compounds that exhibit antispasmodic and anti-inflammatory properties, making it particularly effective in alleviating tightness in the chest and easing coughs. Its action on the respiratory system helps reduce irritation in the airways, allowing for smoother breathing. Studies suggest that grindelia may support lung function by assisting in the expulsion of mucus, thereby promoting clearer airways.

Most Potent Method of Ingestion

The most effective way to utilize grindelia is through an herbal extract or syrup, because these forms preserve the plant's therapeutic properties while providing soothing relief. A well-prepared extract can be taken directly or mixed with warm water or honey to enhance its flavor and effectiveness.

Simple Recipe: Grindelia Syrup

Combine 1 cup of fresh grindelia leaves with 2 cups of water. Simmer for 30 minutes, strain, and add honey to taste. Store in a cool place and take 1 tablespoon as needed to relieve coughs and promote open airways.

Best Herbs to Use Together

When combined with thyme or marshmallow root, grindelia's effects are amplified, creating a powerful respiratory support blend that helps soothe irritation and promote clearer breathing.

RELIEF FROM ASTHMA SYMPTOMS

33. Coleus (*Coleus forskohlii*)

Historical Context

In traditional Ayurvedic medicine, coleus has long been used for its remarkable ability to support respiratory health. In Southeast Asia, it was known as "pungent mint" for curing various ailments, particularly those affecting the lungs. The roots of this hardy plant are often brewed into teas or tinctures.

Active Compounds and Benefits

The star of coleus is forskolin, a potent compound that acts on the smooth muscle of the bronchial passages. Forskolin promotes relaxation and dilation of these muscles, facilitating easier airflow and relieving asthma symptoms. This action makes coleus a powerful ally for individuals struggling with wheezing, shortness of breath, or other respiratory issues. Additionally, coleus enhances the body's ability to respond to allergens, further supporting lung health.

Most Potent Method of Ingestion

Coleus is most effective when consumed as a tincture or in capsule form. The tincture, made from fresh roots, allows for quick absorption and can be taken several times a day for optimal effects. Alternatively, a standardized extract in capsule form provides a convenient option for those seeking consistent doses.

Simple Recipe: Coleus Tea

Steep 1 teaspoon of dried coleus leaves in a cup of hot water for 10–15 minutes. Strain, and sweeten with honey if desired. This soothing tea can be enjoyed daily to support respiratory function and ease asthma symptoms.

Best Herbs to Use Together

Combining coleus with ginger or turmeric creates a powerful synergy that enhances anti-inflammatory effects. Together, these herbs can help nurture and strengthen lung health.

34. Butterbur (*Petasites hybridus*)

Historical Context

This herb was once valued by ancient herbalists and had roots in traditional European medicine. Known for its large, heart-shaped leaves, butterbur has been used for centuries to alleviate discomfort associated with allergies and respiratory conditions. Its name, derived from its traditional use in butter-making, speaks to its historical significance and versatility as an herbal remedy.

Active Compounds and Benefits

Butterbur contains potent phytochemicals, particularly petasin and isopetasin, which have been shown to reduce spasms in the respiratory system. These compounds act as natural relaxants, easing the tension in bronchial muscles and relieving asthma symptoms. Additionally, butterbur is known for its antihistamine properties, which benefit individuals suffering from allergy-induced asthma.

Most Potent Method of Ingestion

The most effective way to harness butterbur's benefits is through standardized extracts or capsules. These forms ensure a precise dosage, allowing for safe and effective use. Fresh butterbur can also be made into teas, although caution should be exercised due to potential toxicity in raw forms.

Simple Recipe: Butterbur Infusion

Steep 1 teaspoon of dried butterbur leaves in 1 cup of boiling water for 10 minutes. Strain and enjoy warm. This soothing infusion can help relax the airways and ease breathing discomfort.

Best Herbs to Use Together

When paired with peppermint or fennel, butterbur's calming effects are enhanced. This provides a well-rounded approach to managing asthma symptoms and promoting respiratory ease. Together, these herbs work harmoniously to create a supportive blend for lung health.

HERBS FOR RESPIRATORY CONDITIONS

MANAGING ALLERGIES

35. Quercetin (*from various plants*)

Historical Context

Quercetin, a powerful flavonoid found in various fruits, vegetables, and herbs, has been cherished throughout history for its numerous health benefits. Its name derives from the Latin word *quercus*, meaning oak, because it was initially isolated from the bark of oak trees. Traditionally, quercetin has been utilized in folk medicine to combat seasonal allergies, promote cardiovascular health, and provide antioxidant protection. This humble yet potent compound embodies nature's wisdom in enhancing wellness.

Active Compounds and Benefits

As a natural antihistamine, quercetin plays a crucial role in stabilizing mast cells, which release histamine during allergic reactions. By inhibiting this release, quercetin effectively reduces allergy-related respiratory symptoms, such as sneezing, congestion, and itching. Its anti-inflammatory properties also contribute to alleviating airway irritation, making it a valuable ally for individuals suffering from asthma and other respiratory conditions.

Most Potent Method of Ingestion

Quercetin is most effective when consumed as a supplement in capsule or powder form, allowing for precise dosages. Additionally, incorporating quercetin-rich foods into your diet, such as apples, onions, and citrus fruits, can naturally bolster your body's defenses against allergies.

Simple Recipe: Quercetin Smoothie

Blend 1 apple, 1 orange, a handful of spinach, and a tablespoon of honey with a cup of water or plant-based milk. This refreshing smoothie not only delights the palate but also delivers a natural dose of quercetin to help manage allergy symptoms.

Best Herbs to Use Together

When combined with stinging nettle, quercetin's effects are amplified, creating a synergistic blend that offers comprehensive relief from seasonal allergies. Together, they form a powerful duo for nurturing respiratory wellness and restoring balance to the body.

36. Nettle (*Urtica dioica*)

Historical Context

Nettle has held a special place in herbal medicine across various cultures. Known for its fierce sting, this hard plant has been utilized for centuries to treat many ailments, particularly seasonal allergies. The Romans prize the nettle for its refreshing properties, while European herbalists have long recognized its value in alleviatin respiratory discomfort. Today, nettle continues to be a cherished remedy in modern herbalism.

Active Compounds and Benefits

Rich in vitamins, minerals, and phytochemicals, nettle is renowned for its anti-inflammatory an antihistamine properties. It contains compounds that inhibit histamine release, helping to alleviate allergy related respiratory symptoms such as nasal congestion, sneezing, and itchy eyes. Nettle's high levels of vitami C further enhance its effectiveness in supporting immune function, making it a formidable ally during allerg season.

Most Potent Method of Ingestion

Nettle can be consumed in various forms, but herbal infusions and tinctures are particularly effective. The preparations capture the plant's healing essence and make it readily available for the body to absorb.

Simple Recipe: Nettle Tea

Steep 1-2 teaspoons of dried nettle leaves in a cup of boiling water for 10–15 minutes. Strain and add hone or lemon for flavor. Enjoy this nourishing tea daily during allergy season to help soothe respiratory symptom

Best Herbs to Use Together

Nettle enhances overall allergy relief when paired with quercetin-rich foods or supplements. This provides comprehensive approach to managing respiratory discomfort.

PROMOTING LUNG HEALTH

37. Cordyceps (*Cordyceps sinensis*)

Historical Context

Popular in traditional Chinese medicine, Cordyceps has been a symbol of vitality and longevity for centuries. This unique fungus thrives at high altitudes, often found on caterpillar larvae, and has been treasured for its exceptional health benefits. Ancient texts praise its ability to invigorate the spirit and enhance stamina, making it a sought-after remedy among emperors and athletes alike. Today, Cordyceps continues to capture the imagination of herbalists and wellness enthusiasts for its profound effects on respiratory health.

Active Compounds and Benefits

Cordyceps contains bioactive compounds, including cordycepin and polysaccharides, which work harmoniously to enhance lung capacity and overall respiratory function. By increasing oxygen utilization and improving endurance, Cordyceps helps the lungs operate at peak efficiency. Its adaptogenic properties also aid in reducing stress and fatigue, which can significantly impact respiratory health.

Most Potent Method of Ingestion

For optimal results, Cordyceps is best consumed as a concentrated extract or in capsule form. This allows for precise dosing and ensures that the body can effectively absorb its beneficial compounds. Additionally, powdered Cordyceps can be added to smoothies, soups, or herbal teas, integrating this powerful fungus into your daily routine.

Simple Recipe: Cordyceps Smoothie

Blend together 1 banana, 1 tablespoon of Cordyceps powder, a handful of spinach, and a cup of almond milk. This energizing smoothie not only supports lung health but also delights the palate with its creamy texture and natural sweetness.

Best Herbs to Use Together

When paired with yerba santa, Cordyceps creates a harmonious blend that promotes lung vitality and eases respiratory discomfort. Together, these two herbs form a formidable alliance, supporting respiratory resilience and overall well-being.

38. Yerba Santa (*Eriodictyon californicum*)

Historical Context

Yerba santa, known as the "holy herb," has been a cherished remedy among Native American tribes for many years. This aromatic plant has been used traditionally to address respiratory ailments and promote overall lung health. Its name reflects the deep respect and spiritual significance that it holds in herbal medicine.

Active Compounds and Benefits

Yerba santa is rich in flavonoids and essential oils, which contribute to its soothing and expectorant properties. This herb is renowned for promoting healthy lung function and easing respiratory discomfort. By relaxing bronchial passages and reducing inflammation, yerba santa allows for easier breathing and relief from coughs. Its anti-inflammatory effects also support lung tissue health, making it a valuable ally for those with chronic respiratory conditions.

Most Potent Method of Ingestion

For maximum benefit, yerba santa can be consumed as a tea, tincture, or capsule. Herbal infusions capture the essence of this aromatic plant, making it readily available for the body to absorb its healing properties.

Simple Recipe: Yerba Santa Infusion

Steep 1–2 teaspoons of dried yerba santa leaves in a cup of hot water for 10–15 minutes. Strain and sweeten with honey or enjoy it plain. This infusion can be sipped daily to support lung health and relieve respiratory discomfort.

Best Herbs to Use Together

When combined with Cordyceps, yerba santa creates a powerful synergy that enhances lung capacity and promotes respiratory function. Together, they form a holistic approach to nurturing lung health and resilience.

REDUCING SINUS PRESSURE

39. Horseradish (*Armoracia rusticana*)

Historical Context

A hardy perennial with roots steeped in tradition, horseradish has been celebrated since ancient times for its potent medicinal qualities. Originating in Eastern Europe, it was once considered a culinary staple and a remedy for various ailments. This herb has an intense aroma and sharp flavor, and has been used not only to spice up dishes but also to clear nasal passages and provide relief from respiratory discomfort. Its use dates back to the Romans, who revered it for its ability to awaken the senses and invigorate the spirit.

Active Compounds and Benefits

Horseradish's power lies in its active compounds, particularly allyl isothiocyanate, which contributes to its distinctive heat and medicinal properties. This compound helps break down mucus, making it easier to expel, and provides a natural decongestant effect. By stimulating circulation and promoting drainage in the sinuses, horseradish can alleviate the discomfort associated with sinus pressure and congestion, offering a breath of fresh air to those suffering from seasonal allergies or respiratory infections.

Most Potent Method of Ingestion

To harness the full benefits of horseradish, it is best consumed fresh or as a tincture. Grating fresh horseradish root releases its volatile oils, which can be mixed into salads, sauces, or taken as a potent herbal remedy.

Simple Recipe: Horseradish Infusion

Mix 1 tablespoon of freshly grated horseradish root with 1 cup of hot water. Let steep for 10 minutes, strain, and add honey or lemon for taste. This refreshing infusion can clear nasal passages and soothe sinus pressure.

Best Herbs to Use Together

Combining horseradish with bayberry enhances their synergistic effects, offering a powerful remedy for sinus relief. Together, they work to break down mucus and reduce inflammation, promoting clear airways and easier breathing.

40. Bayberry (*Myrica cerifera*)

Historical Context

Bayberry is known for its astringent properties and ability to promote overall respiratory health. Indigenous to North America, the waxy bayberry berries were utilized by Native Americans not only as a food source but also as a remedy for various ailments, particularly for respiratory conditions. The warm, earthy aroma of bayberry evokes a sense of comfort, making it a cherished herb for many generations.

Active Compounds and Benefits

Rich in tannins and flavonoids, bayberry is a powerful astringent that helps reduce mucus buildup and alleviate sinus pressure. Its anti-inflammatory properties support healthy mucous membranes, allowing for clearer breathing. Bayberry can also promote circulation, which aids in expulsing mucus and alleviating sinus discomfort.

Most Potent Method of Ingestion

Bayberry can be consumed in several forms, including tinctures, capsules, and decoctions. Its astringent nature is best harnessed in concentrated forms to maximize its benefits.

Simple Recipe: Bayberry Decoction

Simmer 1 tablespoon of dried bayberry bark in 2 cups of water for 20 minutes. Strain and sweeten with honey if desired. This warming decoction soothes the sinuses and reduces pressure, bringing relief to those feeling congested.

Best Herbs to Use Together

When paired with horseradish, bayberry forms a potent duo that tackles sinus pressure head-on. The combined astringent and decongestant properties work together to restore balance and comfort to the respiratory system.

Want another guide of healing modalities, as a thank you?

Hi! It's Ava again. I'm so glad you're exploring the powerful benefits of herbalism. I hope this book is opening your eyes to the incredible world of natural remedies and inspiring you to incorporate these healing practices into your daily life. Another unique healing modality that complements herbalism beautifully is essential oils.

As a Token of My Appreciation, I'd like to offer you an exclusive 25-page Beginner's Guide to Healing Modalities. This guide is designed to broaden your understanding and application of natural health practices, ensuring you have a well-rounded toolkit at your disposal.

This Guide Contains:

- **Explore essential oils,** how they work, and their impact on your wellbeing.
- **Discover the emotional benefits of essential oils** for stress relief, mood enhancement, and mental clarity.
- **Learn practical tips for integrating essential oils** into your daily routines, morning through night.
- **Find out how to select the right essential oils** tailored to your specific health needs and lifestyle.
- **Use essential oils for physical health**, including pain relief and respiratory care.

If you're interested in exploring the full range of natural healing practices, from essential oils to advanced herbal remedies, scan the QR code or use the link on this page to download your free Beginner's Guide to Healing Modalities. Start your journey to comprehensive wellness today! ...

HERBS FOR
SKIN CONDITIONS

WOUND HEALING

41. Comfrey (*Symphytum officinale*)

Historical Context

Comfrey, often called "knitbone," has been a popular herbal ally throughout the ages. It was known for its remarkable ability to mend wounds and fractures. Ancient Greeks and Romans utilized this resilient plant, applying its poultices to promote rapid healing. Its rich, leafy presence has graced gardens for centuries, while folklore echoes its significance in folk medicine as a symbol of recovery and regeneration.

Active Compounds and Benefits

Comfrey's healing prowess lies in its key active compound, allantoin, which stimulates cell growth and tissue repair. This remarkable herb is also rich in mucilage and tannins, offering soothing and anti-inflammatory benefits that alleviate pain and swelling. When applied topically, comfrey creates a protective barrier, keeping wounds moist and allowing optimal healing while preventing infections. It is a natural bandage, promoting swift recovery for minor cuts and deeper abrasions.

Most Potent Method of Ingestion

For those seeking the most effective use of comfrey, topical applications, such as salves or poultices, are the best choice. Apply fresh comfrey poultice directly to the wound for a few hours daily until healed.

Simple Recipe: Comfrey Healing Poultice

Harvest fresh comfrey leaves and crush them into a paste. Apply the paste directly onto the wound, covering it with a clean cloth. Leave it on for several hours or overnight.

Best Herbs to Use Together

When paired with plantain, comfrey enhances its wound-healing effects. Plantain's anti-inflammatory and antimicrobial properties create a powerful combination that nurtures skin recovery.

42. Plantain (*Plantago major*)

Historical Context

Plantain, often regarded as a humble weed (not to be confused with the plantain banana), has a rich history in herbal medicine, utilized by Indigenous cultures across the globe. Known as "nature's band-aid," this resilient plant has been known for its ability to heal wounds and soothe irritated skin.

Active Compounds and Benefits

Plantain's healing powers stem from its high content of allantoin, tannins, and flavonoids. These compounds work synergistically to reduce inflammation, promote cell regeneration, and alleviate pain. Plantain's anti-inflammatory properties make it especially effective in treating insect bites, minor cuts, and skin irritations.

Most Potent Method of Ingestion

The most effective way to harness the healing properties of plantain is through topical applications, such as fresh poultices or infused oils. Use fresh plantain poultice on the affected area for relief, repeating as necessary throughout the day.

Simple Recipe: Plantain-Infused Oil

Fill a jar with fresh plantain leaves and cover them with olive oil. Seal the jar and let it sit in a sunny spot for 2 weeks, shaking occasionally. Strain the oil and apply as needed.

Best Herbs to Use Together

Plantain and comfrey combine powerfully in wound healing.

SOOTHING ECZEMA AND PSORIASIS

43. Yellow Dock (*Rumex crispus*)

Historical Context

Yellow dock has long been celebrated in herbal traditions for its ability to promote skin health. Native American tribes often utilized its roots for their potential to detoxify the body and soothe skin irritations.

Active Compounds and Benefits

Yellow dock is rich in anthraquinones, tannins, and flavonoids, which contribute to its powerful anti-inflammatory and astringent properties. The high levels of vitamins A and C support skin health by encouraging healing and reducing inflammation associated with conditions like eczema and psoriasis. Yellow dock acts as a natural blood purifier, which can help address underlying issues contributing to skin flare-ups. Its ability to enhance liver function further aids detoxification, promoting clearer skin from within.

Most Potent Method of Ingestion

Yellow dock is most effective when taken as a tincture or infused oil. For internal use, a typical dose of yellow dock tincture is 1–2 teaspoons, taken 1–3 times daily, or as directed by a healthcare provider.

Simple Recipe: Yellow Dock–Infused Oil

Fill a jar with dried yellow dock roots and cover with olive oil. Let it steep in a warm, dark place for 4–6 weeks, shaking occasionally. Strain and apply to affected areas as needed.

Best Herbs to Use Together

Combining yellow dock with evening primrose enhances its skin-soothing effects. Evening primrose oil, rich in gamma-linolenic acid (GLA), works synergistically to reduce inflammation and promote skin barrier function, making this duo a powerful ally against eczema and psoriasis.

44. Evening Primrose (*Oenothera biennis*)

Historical Context

Evening primrose has a storied history. It was cherished by Native American tribes and early European settlers for its therapeutic properties. This delicate yellow flower was traditionally used to soothe various ailments, including skin conditions. Its name reflects the plant's beauty and its evening bloom, symbolizing hope and healing under the night sky.

Active Compounds and Benefits

The primary active compound in evening primrose is gamma-linolenic acid (GLA), an essential fatty acid crucial to maintaining skin health. GLA has anti-inflammatory properties, effectively reducing redness, itching, and irritation associated with eczema and psoriasis. Additionally, evening primrose oil helps to strengthen the skin barrier, preventing moisture loss and enhancing overall hydration. Its ability to regulate inflammatory responses supports healthier skin and alleviates flare-ups.

Most Potent Method of Ingestion

Evening primrose oil is most beneficial when taken in capsule form or applied topically as an oil. The typical dose for evening primrose oil capsules is 500 mg, taken 2–3 times daily or as a healthcare provider recommends.

Simple Recipe: Evening Primrose Oil Skin Salve

Melt 1 ounce of beeswax and mix in 2 ounces of evening primrose oil. Stir until blended and pour into a small container. Allow to cool and apply to affected areas as needed.

Best Herbs to Use Together

When paired with yellow dock, evening primrose amplifies its healing potential. This combination provides a comprehensive approach to addressing eczema and psoriasis, promoting symptom relief and a pathway to long-term skin health and vitality.

HERBS FOR SKIN CONDITIONS

TREATING ACNE

45. Tea Tree (*Melaleuca alternifolia*)

Historical Context

Tea tree oil, derived from the leaves of the *Melaleuca alternifolia* tree, has a history rooted in the Aboriginal cultures of Australia. Indigenous Australians utilized this potent oil for its antimicrobial properties, applying it to wounds and skin infections. The name "tea tree" stems from the use of its leaves to brew a medicinal tea, believed to bolster overall health. Today, tea tree oil is revered globally as a powerful ally in treating acne and promoting clear skin.

Active Compounds and Benefits

The primary active compounds in tea tree oil are terpinen-4-ol and 1,8-cineole, which exhibit remarkable antibacterial and anti-inflammatory properties. This herb effectively combats the bacteria that contribute to acne formation while reducing redness and swelling associated with breakouts. By promoting a balanced complexion and reducing excess oil production, tea tree oil helps prevent future acne flare-ups. Its natural astringent qualities tighten pores, providing a dual action that treats and prevents acne.

Most Potent Method of Ingestion

Tea tree oil is most beneficial when used topically, diluted with a carrier oil, or as part of a skincare regimen. For topical application, a typical dosage involves mixing 1–2 drops of tea tree oil with a carrier oil (such as jojoba or coconut oil) and applying it directly to blemishes once or twice daily.

Simple Recipe: Tea Tree Oil Acne Spot Treatment

Mix 1 drop of tea tree oil with 2 drops of carrier oil. Dab the mixture onto affected areas using a clean cotton swab. Allow to absorb; repeat as needed.

Best Herbs to Use Together

Pairing tea tree oil with holy basil enhances its acne-fighting capabilities. Holy basil is known for its adaptogenic properties and anti-inflammatory effects, supporting the skin's healing process and reducing stress-related breakouts.

46. Holy Basil (*Ocimum sanctum*)

Historical Context

Revered in Ayurvedic medicine, holy basil, or Tulsi, is considered a sacred herb in India. For thousands of years, it has been utilized not just for its culinary flavor but also for its medicinal virtues. Holy basil's rich history in traditional medicine highlights its role as a holistic remedy, balancing mind, body, and spirit while promoting skin health.

Active Compounds and Benefits

Holy basil is abundant in eugenol, rosmarinic acid, and various antioxidants, which contribute to its potent anti-inflammatory and antimicrobial effects. These compounds help reduce acne-causing bacteria, soothe inflamed skin, and mitigate the effects of oxidative stress, making holy basil an excellent remedy for acne-prone skin. Additionally, its adaptogenic properties help the body manage stress, a known trigger for breakouts, promoting a calmer complexion.

Most Potent Method of Ingestion

Holy basil can be consumed as a tea or used in topical formulations for maximum benefit. For internal use, typical dose is 1–2 teaspoons of dried holy basil leaves steeped in hot water, consumed 1–2 times daily. For topical use, holy basil–infused oil can be applied directly to the skin.

Simple Recipe: Holy Basil Tea

Steep 1–2 teaspoons of dried holy basil leaves in a cup of boiling water for 10 minutes. Strain and enjoy sweetened with honey if desired. For topical use, mix infused oil with a few drops of tea tree oil and apply as needed.

Best Herbs to Use Together

When combined with tea tree, holy basil creates a synergistic effect that addresses the root causes of acne while promoting overall skin health. Together, they form a robust duo, tackling blemishes from multiple angles for clearer, healthier skin.

MOISTURIZING DRY SKIN

47. Jojoba (*Simmondsia chinensis*)

Historical Context

Native to the arid landscapes of the American Southwest, jojoba has long been a cherished botanical in traditional Indigenous practices. The seeds of the jojoba plant have been pressed to extract oil for centuries, serving as a natural moisturizer for both skin and hair.

Active Compounds and Benefits

Jojoba oil is unique in its composition, closely resembling human sebum, the natural oil that your skin produces. Rich in fatty acids, vitamins E and B, and antioxidants, it penetrates the skin effortlessly, providing deep hydration without clogging pores. Jojoba moisturizes and helps balance oil production, making it suitable for all skin types. Its anti-inflammatory properties soothe irritated skin and promote a healthier complexion, while its antimicrobial qualities help protect against skin infections.

Most Potent Method of Ingestion

Jojoba is best used topically as a pure oil or incorporated into skincare products. To moisturize dry skin, apply 1–2 drops of jojoba oil directly onto clean skin, massaging gently until fully absorbed.

Simple Recipe: Jojoba Hydrating Serum

Combine 2 tablespoons of jojoba oil with 5 drops of essential oil (such as lavender or frankincense) in a small bottle. Shake gently to mix. Apply a few drops to the face and neck daily for intense hydration.

Best Herbs to Use Together

Pairing jojoba with olive oil enhances its moisturizing benefits. Olive oil, rich in antioxidants and fatty acids, complements jojoba's nourishing properties, creating a powerful blend for combating dryness.

48. Olive Oil (*Olea europaea*)

Historical Context

Since ancient times, olive oil has been a staple in Mediterranean diets and a symbol of health and prosperity. Known as "liquid gold," it has played a significant role in traditional medicine, beauty rituals, and culinary arts. The ancient Greeks and Romans valued olive oil not only for its nutritional benefits but also for its skin-nourishing properties, using it to moisturize and protect their skin from harsh elements.

Active Compounds and Benefits

Olive oil is abundant in monounsaturated fats, antioxidants, and vitamins A and E, which provide deep hydration and promote skin elasticity. Its emollient properties create a protective barrier on the skin, locking in moisture and preventing dryness. The oleic acid found in olive oil enhances skin absorption, delivering nutrients directly to where needed. Additionally, its anti-inflammatory effects help soothe irritated skin, making it an excellent remedy for conditions like eczema and psoriasis.

Most Potent Method of Ingestion

Olive oil is most effective when used topically or incorporated into daily diets. For topical application, use 1-2 teaspoons of olive oil on clean skin or mix with other ingredients in skincare formulations.

Simple Recipe: Olive Oil and Sugar Scrub

Mix 1 tablespoon of olive oil with 2 tablespoons of sugar in a small bowl. Gently exfoliate the skin in circular motions before rinsing with warm water. Pat dry and follow with a moisturizer.

Best Herbs to Use Together

When combined with jojoba, olive oil enhances the hydrating effects, creating a synergistic blend that revitalizes dry skin and restores its natural glow.

RELIEVING BURNS AND SUNBURNS

49. Aloe Vera (*Aloe barbadensis*)

Historical Context

Aloe vera, often referred to as the "plant of immortality," has been revered for centuries. In ancient Egypt, it was used for its healing properties. This succulent has been a staple in traditional medicine across various cultures, from the Chinese to the Greeks, celebrated for its ability to soothe and heal skin ailments. Its gel-like sap, often associated with beauty and wellness, symbolizes nature's gentle touch in times of need.

Active Compounds and Benefits

The leaves of the aloe vera plant are packed with vitamins, enzymes, amino acids, and polysaccharides, all contributing to its remarkable healing abilities. Aloe vera's cooling properties provide instant relief from burns and sunburns, reducing redness and inflammation. The gel is also known to promote skin regeneration, helping to repair damaged tissue and restore the skin's moisture barrier. Its antibacterial properties prevent infection, making it an essential remedy for minor wounds and sunburns.

Most Potent Method of Ingestion

Aloe vera is most effective when applied topically in its pure gel form, allowing for maximum absorption and relief. For optimal soothing effects, apply generous amounts of fresh aloe vera gel directly to the affected area 2–3 times daily.

Simple Recipe: Soothing Aloe Vera Gel

Cut a fresh aloe vera leaf and scoop out the gel using a spoon. Make sure to scoop the gel and not the yellow latex layer just inside the skin, which has toxic properties. Apply the gel directly to sunburned or burned skin, massaging gently. Store any unused gel in a sealed container in the refrigerator for future use.

Best Herbs to Use Together

When paired with mallow, aloe vera's soothing effects are amplified. Mallow's mucilage-rich leaves further enhance the calming properties, providing a double layer of relief for irritated skin.

50. Mallow (*Malva sylvestris*)

Historical Context

Known as a wildflower with a rich history, common mallow (known as "Cheeses" and not to be confused with marshmallow) has been cherished since ancient times for its culinary and medicinal uses. The Greeks and Romans utilized mallow for its soothing qualities. With its vibrant pink flowers and delicate leaves, mallow symbolizes nourishment and care, embodying nature's gentle embrace in healing.

Active Compounds and Benefits

Mallow is renowned for its high mucilage content, which provides a protective, soothing layer on the skin. This herb contains flavonoids and tannins, known for their anti-inflammatory properties. Mallow's gentle nature makes it ideal for calming burns, rashes, and sunburns, reducing pain and promoting healing. Its hydrating qualities help maintain skin moisture.

Most Potent Method of Ingestion

Mallow is best used as a poultice or infusion to harness its soothing benefits effectively. For topical application, apply a mallow poultice to the affected area as needed.

Simple Recipe: Mallow Infusion

Steep 1 tablespoon of dried mallow leaves in a cup of hot water for 10–15 minutes. Strain and allow to cool. Use the infusion to soak a clean cloth and apply it to burns or sunburns for relief.

Best Herbs to Use Together

When combined with aloe vera, mallow enhances the soothing effect, creating a nurturing remedy that cools and heals, restoring skin health after burns and sun exposure.

REDUCING SCARRING

51. Rosehip Seed Oil (*from Rosa canina*)

Historical Context

Rosehip seed oil, derived from the seeds of wild rose bushes, has been a treasured beauty secret for centuries. Used by Indigenous peoples of South America and later embraced by European herbalists, it was revered for its skin-nourishing properties. This oil has often been referred to as "nature's scar healer," embodying the spirit of regeneration found in the wild rose.

Active Compounds and Benefits

Rich in essential fatty acids, antioxidants, and vitamins A and C, rosehip seed oil possesses remarkable skin-repairing qualities. The oil's high concentration of linoleic and linolenic acids promotes cellular regeneration and enhances skin elasticity, effectively minimizing the appearance of scars and hyperpigmentation. Its natural anti-inflammatory properties help soothe irritation and redness, promoting an even skin tone. Additionally, the antioxidants protect against environmental damage.

Most Potent Method of Ingestion

The oil is best used topically—direct application on scars to maximize its healing benefits. Apply a few drops of rosehip seed oil directly to the scarred area twice daily, gently massaging it into the skin for optimal absorption.

Simple Recipe: Rosehip Scar Serum

Combine 2 tablespoons of rosehip seed oil with 1 tablespoon of vitamin E oil in a small glass dropper bottle. Shake gently to mix. Apply to scars morning and night for enhanced healing.

Best Herbs to Use Together

Rosehip seed oil creates a powerful synergy when blended with myrrh. Myrrh's antiseptic and anti-inflammatory properties complement rosehip oil, enhancing scar reduction quality.

52. Myrrh (*Commiphora myrrha*)

Historical Context

Myrrh, a resin obtained from the *Commiphora* tree, has been used in ancient times for its aromatic and medicinal properties. In Egyptian embalming rituals, it was used as a precious ingredient in incense. Myrrh symbolizes healing and purification.

Active Compounds and Benefits

Myrrh contains active compounds such as terpenoids and sesquiterpenes, known for their anti-inflammatory and antimicrobial effects. This resin promotes wound healing and reduces inflammation, making it a valuable ally in scar treatment. Myrrh enhances blood circulation to the skin, facilitating the regeneration of new tissue while preventing infection. Its natural astringent properties help tighten and tone the skin, further minimizing the appearance of scars.

Most Potent Method of Ingestion

Myrrh is most effective when used as an essential oil or infused in carrier oils for topical application. Dilute 2–3 drops of myrrh essential oil in a carrier oil (like jojoba or coconut oil) and apply it to scars once daily.

Simple Recipe: Myrrh-Infused Oil

Combine 1 teaspoon of myrrh resin with 2 tablespoons of carrier oil in a small jar. Allow it to infuse for 1–2 weeks in a warm, dark place. Strain and use the infused oil to massage into scarred areas.

Best Herbs to Use Together

When paired with rosehip seed oil, myrrh enhances the oil's regenerative properties, creating a potent scar reduction remedy that nourishes the skin.

MANAGING FUNGAL INFECTIONS

53. Pau d'Arco (*Tabebuia impetiginosa*)

Historical Context

Pau d'Arco, a majestic tree native to the rainforests of South America, has long been revered for its medicinal properties among Indigenous tribes. Known as "Taheebo" or "Ipe Roxo," its bark has been used for centuries as a potent remedy for various ailments, particularly fungal infections. With its striking purple flowers, this vibrant tree symbolizes resilience and healing, embodying the spirit of nature's bounty in the fight against illness.

Active Compounds and Benefits

Pau d'Arco contains a unique compound called "lapachol," which exhibits strong antifungal, antibacterial, and anti-inflammatory properties. This natural remedy works by inhibiting the growth of fungi, making it particularly effective in treating infections such as *Candida* and athlete's foot. Its immune-boosting properties further support the body in combating infections, promoting overall wellness. Pau d'Arco is also known for its detoxifying effects, helping to cleanse the body of harmful pathogens.

Most Potent Method of Ingestion

For optimal results, Pau d'Arco is best consumed as a tea or tincture, allowing for the extraction of its powerful active compounds. When taken as a tea, drink 1–2 cups daily. For tincture form, take 30–40 drops diluted in water twice a day.

Simple Recipe: Pau d'Arco Tea

Add 1–2 teaspoons of dried Pau d'Arco bark to a cup of boiling water. Let it steep for 10–15 minutes.

Strain and enjoy, adding honey or lemon to taste if desired.

Best Herbs to Use Together

Combining Pau d'Arco with clove enhances its antifungal properties. Together, they create a formidable duo against fungal infections, amplifying the body's natural defenses.

54. Clove (*Syzygium aromaticum*)

Historical Context

Clove, derived from the flower buds of the clove tree, has been treasured for centuries in traditional medicine and culinary practices. Revered in ancient Chinese and Indian cultures, it was a highly sought-after spice in the spice trade, symbolizing wealth and luxury. With its rich history as a remedy for various ailments, clove has stood the test of time.

Active Compounds and Benefits

Clove is rich in eugenol, a potent compound known for its antifungal, antibacterial, and analgesic properties. This powerful ingredient makes clove an effective treatment for fungal infections, inhibiting the growth of pathogens while soothing inflammation. Its antioxidant properties further protect the skin from damage, while its ability to promote blood circulation enhances overall skin health. Clove also helps relieve pain and discomfort associated with fungal infections.

Most Potent Method of Ingestion

Clove is most effective when used as an essential oil or in powdered form, either in teas or topical applications. For topical use, dilute 2–3 drops of clove essential oil in a carrier oil and apply it to the affected area once a day. For internal use, consume 1–2 teaspoons of powdered clove in warm water or food.

Simple Recipe: Clove Infusion

Boil 1 cup of water and add 1 teaspoon of whole cloves. Let it steep for 10–15 minutes. Strain and enjoy as a soothing beverage.

Best Herbs to Use Together

When paired with Pau d'Arco, clove enhances the antifungal effects, creating a potent natural remedy that combats fungal infections effectively and supports skin health.

REDUCING REDNESS AND SWELLING

55. Witch Hazel (*Hamamelis virginiana*)

Historical Context

Witch hazel, a beloved native shrub of North America, has been a staple in herbal medicine for centuries. Native Americans recognized its soothing properties, using the bark and leaves in poultices to treat inflammation, wounds, and skin irritations. The name "witch hazel" derives from the Old English term "wiche," meaning "to bend," referring to the plant's pliable branches.

Active Compounds and Benefits

Witch hazel is rich in tannins and flavonoids, which contribute to its anti-inflammatory and astringent properties. These compounds help reduce swelling and redness, making witch hazel a go-to remedy for conditions such as acne, rosacea, and minor skin irritations. Its natural astringency tightens the skin and minimizes the appearance of pores, promoting a clear and healthy complexion. Additionally, witch hazel provides relief from itching and discomfort, soothing sensitive skin.

Most Potent Method of Ingestion

The most effective way to utilize witch hazel is through topical application as a liquid extract or infused in creams and ointments. For external use, apply witch hazel extract directly to the affected area with a cotton ball 1–2 times daily.

Simple Recipe: Witch Hazel Soothing Compress

Soak a clean cloth in witch hazel extract. Apply it to the irritated area for 10–15 minutes. Repeat as needed to soothe redness and swelling.

Best Herbs to Use Together

Witch hazel and St. John's Wort combine powerfully to enhance their soothing effects on inflamed skin. Together, they provide comprehensive relief from redness and irritation, promoting a calmer complexion.

56. St. John's Wort (*Hypericum perforatum*)

Historical Context

St. John's Wort, known for its bright yellow flowers and legendary healing properties, has been utilized since ancient times. Historically, this herb was named after St. John the Baptist, because it often blooms around his feast day in June. Traditional cultures have celebrated its use for a variety of ailments, particularly for its mood-enhancing effects and ability to soothe the skin. This herbal remedy represents the union of nature and spirituality, embodying the power of botanical healing.

Active Compounds and Benefits

The key active compounds in St. John's Wort include hypericin and hyperforin, which possess potent anti-inflammatory and analgesic properties. This herb is renowned for its ability to reduce redness and swelling, making it an ideal choice for conditions such as eczema and psoriasis. St. John's Wort also promotes skin healing by stimulating tissue regeneration, providing relief from irritation and discomfort while enhancing the skin's overall appearance.

Most Potent Method of Ingestion

St. John's Wort is most effective when used topically in oils or ointments, although it can also be consumed as a tea. For topical application, apply St. John's Wort oil to the affected area up to twice daily. For tea, steep 1–2 teaspoons of dried flowers in hot water for 10 minutes and drink 1–2 cups daily.

Simple Recipe: St. John's Wort–Infused Oil

Place dried St. John's Wort flowers in a jar and cover with olive oil. Seal and let it sit in a warm place for 4–6 weeks, shaking occasionally. Strain and store in a dark bottle for topical use.

Best Herbs to Use Together

When combined with witch hazel, St. John's Wort enhances its anti-inflammatory effects, providing a dual action approach to reduce redness and swelling while promoting skin health.

PROMOTING A HEALTHY SKIN BARRIER

57. Cocoa Butter (*from Theobroma cacao seeds*)

Historical Context

Cocoa butter, derived from the seeds of the cacao tree, traces its roots back to the ancient civilizations of Mesoamerica. The Aztecs and Mayans revered cacao not only as a source of nourishment but also as a sacred substance, and they used it in rituals and as currency. This rich, creamy fat has since evolved into a beloved ingredient in skincare, celebrated for its ability to hydrate and protect the skin. Its legacy symbolizes luxury and self-care, deeply intertwined with beauty traditions.

Active Compounds and Benefits

Cocoa butter is packed with antioxidants, fatty acids, and vitamins E and K, synergistically promoting skin health. Its high stearic acid content provides a protective barrier against environmental aggressors, helping to lock in moisture and prevent dehydration. This natural emollient is especially beneficial for dry and sensitive skin, reducing irritation while improving elasticity. Its soothing properties also aid in healing scars and stretch marks.

Most Potent Method of Ingestion

While cocoa butter is primarily used topically, it can also be incorporated into skincare formulations such as balms, creams, and lotions for maximum effect. For topical application, apply a small amount of cocoa butter directly to the skin as needed, particularly after bathing, to seal in moisture.

Simple Recipe: Cocoa Butter Moisturizing Balm

Melt 1 cup of cocoa butter in a double boiler. Add 2 tablespoons of coconut oil and stir until combined. Pour into a jar and let cool. Apply as needed to dry areas.

Best Herbs to Use Together

When paired with borage seed oil, cocoa butter's hydrating properties are enhanced, creating a potent blend that supports skin barrier function and nourishes the skin deeply.

58. Borage Seed Oil (*from Borago officinalis*)

Historical Context

Borage, often referred to as the "starflower," has a storied past, dating back to ancient Roman times when was used to promote courage and strength. Historically, herbalists recognized borage for its cooling properties and ability to relieve stress and anxiety. Today, this herb is celebrated for its vibrant blue flowers and nourishing oil, which has become a staple in modern skincare.

Active Compounds and Benefits

Rich in gamma-linolenic acid (GLA), borage seed oil possesses exceptional anti-inflammatory properties that help soothe irritated skin and promote a healthy barrier. Its high fatty acid content aids in moisture retention, making it particularly beneficial for dry and sensitive skin conditions. Borage oil supports skin elasticity and resilience, while its antioxidant properties protect against environmental damage, ensuring a vibrant and youthful complexion.

Most Potent Method of Ingestion

Borage seed oil is best utilized topically, either as a standalone oil or incorporated into creams and lotions. Apply 1–2 drops of borage seed oil directly to the skin or mix with a carrier oil for topical use.

Simple Recipe: Borage Oil-Infused Moisturizer

Combine 1 tablespoon of borage seed oil with 2 tablespoons of aloe vera gel. Mix thoroughly and apply to the skin to hydrate and soothe.

Best Herbs to Use Together

When used with cocoa butter, borage seed oil enhances the moisturizing and protective properties, creating a luxurious blend that nurtures the skin barrier and promotes overall skin health.

DETOXIFYING THE SKIN

59. Celandine (*Chelidonium majus*)

Historical Context
Celandine, often referred to as the "greater celandine," has a rich history steeped in herbal tradition, used since ancient times by the Greeks and Romans for its therapeutic properties. It was valued not only for its vibrant yellow sap but also for its ability to promote overall health. In folklore, celandine was associated with healing, symbolizing renewal and the power of nature to cleanse and rejuvenate the body. Today, this humble plant continues to be recognized for its detoxifying properties.

Active Compounds and Benefits
The active compounds in celandine, including the alkaloids chelidonine and sanguinarine, possess potent anti-inflammatory and antimicrobial properties. This herb is known for its ability to support liver function, assisting in the elimination of toxins from the body. When applied topically, celandine can help to clear skin blemishes and promote a radiant complexion, acting as a natural remedy for conditions such as eczema and psoriasis.

Most Potent Method of Ingestion
Celandine is most effective when used as an infusion or tincture, allowing the body to absorb its healing properties internally. For detoxification, take 1–2 teaspoons of celandine tincture diluted in water once or twice daily. Topically, apply a diluted infusion to affected skin areas.

Simple Recipe: Celandine Infusion
Steep 1 tablespoon of dried celandine in 2 cups of hot water for 10–15 minutes. Strain and cool. Use as a wash for irritated skin or as a detoxifying beverage.

Best Herbs to Use Together
When combined with burdock root, celandine creates a powerful detoxifying synergy that enhances the body's natural cleansing processes and promotes clear skin.

60. Burdock Root (*Arctium lappa*)

Historical Context

Burdock root has a long-standing reputation in traditional herbal medicine, particularly within Chinese and Native American cultures. Revered for its health benefits, burdock was often used as a blood purifier and for treating various skin ailments. Its name derives from the prickly burrs that cling to clothing, symbolizing its tenacity and resilience. Today, burdock is celebrated for its detoxifying properties, serving as a natural remedy for promoting skin health and overall well-being.

Active Compounds and Benefits

Rich in antioxidants, vitamins, and inulin, burdock root acts as a potent detoxifier, promoting liver and kidney health. Its anti-inflammatory properties help soothe irritated skin, while its antibacterial effects make it effective in treating acne and other skin conditions. By supporting the body's elimination pathways, burdock aids in purifying the blood, resulting in a clearer complexion and healthier skin.

Most Potent Method of Ingestion

Burdock root is best consumed as a tea, tincture, or added to soups and stews. For detoxifying benefits, drink 1–2 cups of burdock root tea daily or take 1–2 teaspoons of tincture diluted in water.

Simple Recipe: Burdock Root Tea

Slice 1–2 inches of fresh burdock root and simmer in 4 cups of water for 20 minutes. Strain and enjoy warm or chilled for a refreshing detoxifying drink.

Best Herbs to Use Together

When paired with celandine, burdock root enhances detoxification, creating a harmonious blend that supports skin health and overall vitality.

HERBS FOR
STRESS AND ANXIETY

CALMING THE NERVOUS SYSTEM

61. Skullcap (*Scutellaria lateriflora*)

Historical Context

Skullcap, often called the "mad-dog herb," has a legacy rooted in the early American herbal traditions where it was cherished for its calming influence. European settlers later adopted it for its ability to bring peace to a restless mind and soothe frazzled nerves. This humble, lavender-flowered herb was often brewed as a tea to alleviate tension. Today, skullcap continues to be celebrated as a natural balm for the nervous system.

Active Compounds and Benefits

Rich in flavonoids and phenolic acids, skullcap is particularly high in baicalin, an active compound known for its anxiolytic and anti-inflammatory properties. These compounds work together to ease tension, relax muscles, and reduce feelings of overwhelm. Skullcap's calming effects are also thought to support healthy levels of gamma-aminobutyric acid (GABA), a neurotransmitter that promotes relaxation, making it an ideal herb for individuals who struggle with nervousness or mild anxiety.

Most Potent Method of Ingestion

Skullcap is most effective when taken as a tea or tincture. Its active compounds are gently extracted in water or alcohol, allowing for quick absorption and a soothing effect that permeates both mind and body. For daily calm, take 1–2 teaspoons of skullcap tincture in water once or twice a day. Alternatively, brew skullcap tea and sip as needed.

Simple Recipe: Skullcap Tea for Tranquility

Steep 1 tablespoon of dried skullcap in 1–2 cups of boiling water for 10–15 minutes. Strain, allow to cool slightly, and enjoy the gentle, earthy flavors that bring peace to the spirit and calm to the mind.

Best Herbs to Use Together

Pair skullcap with lemon balm for a deeper relaxation effect. Together, they create a harmonious blend that enhances mental clarity while soothing the nervous system.

62. Passionflower (*Passiflora incarnata*)

Historical Context

Passionflower, a tendrilled beauty with vibrant, unique blooms, has captured the admiration of herbalists and healers for centuries. Indigenous peoples of the Americas first used this vine for its calming qualities, and European settlers soon embraced it as a remedy for easing mental and physical stress. The name "passionflower" stems from Spanish missionaries who saw symbols of Christ's crucifixion in its blossoms, associating it with hope and spiritual resilience.

Active Compounds and Benefits

Passionflower contains alkaloids, flavonoids, and the amino acid gamma-aminobutyric acid (GABA), which work in harmony to calm the mind and ease anxious thoughts. The flavonoid apigenin is particularly effective at reducing stress responses, while GABA's natural sedative effects create a gentle but powerful sense of relaxation.

Most Potent Method of Ingestion

For optimal results, passionflower is best consumed as a tea or tincture. For calming effects, take 1–2 teaspoons of passionflower tincture in a glass of water up to twice a day. Alternatively, brew passionflower tea and sip as needed.

Simple Recipe: Passionflower Calming Tea

Steep 1–2 teaspoons of dried passionflower in a cup of hot water for 10–15 minutes. Strain and enjoy this floral, tranquil brew in moments when the mind and spirit need grounding.

Best Herbs to Use Together

Passionflower blends beautifully with hops for a powerful relaxation effect. This duo works synergistically to calm the nervous system, and ease tension.

SUPPORTING SLEEP

63. Valerian Root (*Valeriana officinalis*)

Historical Context

Valerian root, often called "nature's tranquilizer," has a legacy as ancient as it is profound. It was popular in ancient Greece and Rome for its calming effects since the time of Hippocrates. During medieval times, valerian was known as "heal-all," offering solace to restless souls and sleepless nights. From the opulent halls of Roman emperors to humble folk remedies in medieval Europe, valerian has been a steadfast ally for those searching for restful slumber. Today, this earthy root remains a powerful natural sedative.

Active Compounds and Benefits

The primary compounds in valerian include valerenic acid and isovaleric acid, both of which increase the availability of gamma-aminobutyric acid (GABA) in the brain. This neurotransmitter slows neural activity, reducing stress and promoting relaxation. Additionally, valerian's sesquiterpenes further enhance its tranquil effects, making it especially useful for calming the mind and soothing anxiety before bedtime.

Most Potent Method of Ingestion

Valerian root is most effective when taken as a tincture or in capsule form, because its concentrated active compounds can be quickly absorbed. Valerian tea is another potent option, although its strong, earthy taste may not suit everyone. For restful sleep, take 1–2 teaspoons of valerian tincture about 30 minutes before bed or prepare a tea (see the recipe below).

Simple Recipe: Valerian Sleep Tea

Steep 1 teaspoon of dried valerian root in 1 cup of hot water for 10–15 minutes. Strain and sip slowly before bed.

Best Herbs to Use Together

Combine valerian with lemon balm for a synergistic effect that enhances relaxation.

64. California Poppy (*Eschscholzia californica*)

Historical Context

Known as the Golden State's flower, California poppy has long graced the fields and coasts of North America with its vibrant orange petals. Native tribes revered this beautiful bloom for its gentle sedative properties, using it as a remedy to calm nerves and lull the body into sleep. Unlike the opium poppy, California poppy has no narcotic effect, making it a gentle choice for promoting rest without risk of dependency.

Active Compounds and Benefits

California poppy contains alkaloids like protopine and allocryptopine, which are known to have mild sedative and anti-anxiety effects. Additionally, its antioxidant properties help reduce oxidative stress.

Most Potent Method of Ingestion

For best results, California poppy is most often taken as a tincture or tea. The tincture provides a quick, gentle onset of relaxation, making it an ideal choice for calming the body before bed. For sleep support, take 1–2 teaspoons of California poppy tincture in water about 30 minutes before bed, or brew a tea (see recipe below).

Simple Recipe: California Poppy Bedtime Brew

Steep 1–2 teaspoons of dried California poppy in a cup of hot water for 10 minutes. Strain and enjoy the gentle warmth and tranquility of this soothing bedtime tea.

Best Herbs to Use Together

California poppy pairs harmoniously with chamomile for a gentle, calming blend that helps ease the body into sleep.

BALANCING MOOD

65. Ashwagandha (*Withania somnifera*)

Historical Context

For over 3,000 years, ashwagandha has been revered in Ayurvedic medicine as a rasayana, or rejuvenating herb. Often called the "strength of the stallion," it has a rich history of use to bolster resilience and vitality in times of physical and emotional stress. Ancient Indian texts celebrate this root as an adaptogen that calms and strengthens, restoring harmony to both body and mind. Today, ashwagandha remains a favored choice for balancing mood.

Active Compounds and Benefits

Ashwagandha's key compounds, withanolides, offer a calming effect on the nervous system, lowering cortisol levels and enhancing the body's resistance to stress. The alkaloid somniferine also contributes to its soothing properties, easing anxiety while supporting balanced mood. Ashwagandha's adaptogenic qualities make it particularly powerful for those experiencing stress-induced mood imbalances.

Most Potent Method of Ingestion

Ashwagandha is most effective when taken as a powdered supplement or tincture, which enables easy absorption of its active compounds. To support mood balance, take 1 teaspoon of ashwagandha powder or 1–2 teaspoons of tincture daily.

Simple Recipe: Ashwagandha Mood Balancing Tonic

Add 1 teaspoon of ashwagandha powder to 1 cup of warm milk (or milk alternative). Stir in honey or cinnamon to taste and sip in the evening for a soothing effect.

Best Herbs to Use Together

When paired with holy basil, ashwagandha offers a synergy that enhances emotional resilience.

66. Rhodiola (*Rhodiola rosea*)

Historical Context

Known as the "golden root," rhodiola has been treasured in traditional Russian and Scandinavian medicine for centuries, especially by those in harsh northern climates. Viking warriors historically used this hardy plant to enhance mental and physical endurance. Today, rhodiola is recognized worldwide as an adaptogen that naturally supports emotional balance.

Active Compounds and Benefits

Rhodiola's primary compounds, rosavin and salidroside, contribute to its adaptogenic qualities. They help regulate serotonin and dopamine levels, which are essential for mood regulation. Additionally, their ability to support adrenal function helps prevent burnout and enhance a steady, uplifted mood.

Most Potent Method of Ingestion

Rhodiola is most effective in capsule or tincture form, both of which offer consistent dosing and quick absorption of its active compounds. For mood support, take 200–400 mg of rhodiola extract daily or 1–2 teaspoons of tincture. Start with a lower dose to gauge your response, because rhodiola can have an energizing effect.

Simple Recipe: Rhodiola Energizing Tea

Steep 1 teaspoon of rhodiola root powder in 1 cup of hot water for 10 minutes. Strain and enjoy this energizing tea in the morning to support a balanced, resilient mood.

Best Herbs to Use Together

Rhodiola pairs well with lemon balm to provide a mood-lifting and calming effect.

REDUCING PHYSICAL SYMPTOMS OF ANXIETY

67. Kava (*Piper methysticum*)

Historical Context

Known to the Pacific Islanders as a plant of friendship and peace, kava was historically consumed during gatherings to foster connection and ease interpersonal tensions. This sacred root was believed to hold the spirit of tranquility, and its role in cultural rituals reflects its capacity to unify and calm.

Active Compounds and Benefits

Kava's power lies in its kavalactones, a group of compounds that act on the brain's limbic system—the area responsible for emotions. These kavalactones can effectively relax muscles and reduce the physical symptoms of anxiety, such as tightness, restlessness, and physical discomfort. Kava works by promoting feelings of relaxation without impairing mental clarity, which makes it a favored natural remedy for managing social or performance-related anxiety.

Most Potent Method of Ingestion

Kava is most effective when prepared as a traditional beverage or a tincture. Its calming effects are quickly noticeable. For stress relief, mix 1 teaspoon of powdered kava in water and drink 1–2 times daily, particularly before high-stress situations. Due to potential side effects, limit prolonged use.

Simple Recipe: Kava-Calming Drink

Combine 1 teaspoon of kava powder with 8 ounces of warm water. Let it steep for 10–15 minutes, then strain. Enjoy slowly, savoring the calming effects as they set in.

Best Herbs to Use Together

Pairing kava with chamomile creates a gentle synergy that soothes both mind and body, enhancing relaxation and easing the physical manifestations of stress.

68. Lemon Verbena (*Aloysia citrodora*)

Historical Context

Known for its citrusy aroma, lemon verbena has been cherished in Europe since the 17th century as a calming and uplifting herb. Initially cultivated as an ornamental plant, it soon found its way into apothecaries for its reputation as a "joy herb" that could uplift the spirit and calm frayed nerves. The plant's lemony fragrance was believed to bring mental clarity and ease physical tension.

Active Compounds and Benefits

Lemon verbena's benefits come from its essential oils, particularly citral and limonene, which have muscle-relaxing and anti-anxiety properties. This herb is known to reduce nervous tension and soothe anxiety-associated digestive discomfort. The gentle sedative effects of lemon verbena make it especially beneficial for individuals who experience physical manifestations of anxiety, such as stomach knots and muscle tightness.

Most Potent Method of Ingestion

Lemon verbena works best as a tea, allowing the aromatic oils to release and calm the mind and body, easing mental and physical tension. Steep 1 teaspoon of dried lemon verbena leaves in hot water and drink 2–3 times daily, particularly after meals, to calm anxiety-related physical discomfort.

Simple Recipe: Lemon Verbena Calming Tea

Steep 1 teaspoon of dried lemon verbena in 1 cup of hot water for 5–10 minutes. Strain and enjoy warm, savoring the soothing aroma and taste.

Best Herbs to Use Together

When combined with lavender, lemon verbena enhances its muscle-relaxing and mood-lifting effects, providing an ideal remedy for easing both emotional and physical signs of anxiety.

SUPPORTING ADRENAL HEALTH

69. Ginseng (*Panax ginseng*)

Historical Context

Ginseng, or "the root of life," is celebrated for its ability to reinvigorate both body and mind. Traditional Chinese medicine has long praised this herb as an adaptogen that enhances resilience to physical and mental stress, and its enduring reputation for vitality-boosting properties remains unchanged. Stories of warriors and scholars alike tell of Ginseng's invigorating power, treasured in times of challenge and fatigue.

Active Compounds and Benefits

Ginsenosides, the unique compounds in Ginseng, lend potent adaptogenic qualities that nurture the adrenal glands, regulate cortisol, and support sustained energy. Additionally, Ginseng enhances circulation and immune health, making it a multifaceted ally in stress relief. The herb's influence on hormonal balance further allows it to soothe nervous system tension, ultimately helping the body achieve equilibrium.

Most Potent Method of Ingestion

Ginseng's benefits are well-extracted through tinctures, which preserve its active compounds and promote quick absorption. Capsules offer a convenient alternative, allowing a steady, easy-to-digest release of Ginsenosides for long-term adrenal support. A daily tincture dose of 20–30 drops, taken up to twice a day, can sustain energy and support adrenal health. For capsules, 200–400 mg daily is recommended.

Simple Recipe: Ginseng Tincture

Add 1 ounce of dried Ginseng root to a clean glass jar. Cover with 80–100 proof vodka, ensuring that all root material is submerged. Seal and store in a dark place, shaking daily for 6 weeks. Strain, then take 20 drops as needed.

Best Herbs to Use Together

Ginseng combines well with rhodiola to boost adrenal resilience, while holy basil further complements its stress-moderating properties.

70. Shatavari (*Asparagus racemosus*)

Historical Context

Shatavari, meaning "she who possesses a hundred husbands," has been a cornerstone of Ayurvedic tradition, symbolizing vitality, endurance, and balance. Used primarily to nourish female reproductive health, Shatavari also excels in supporting overall hormonal harmony and adrenal function, a prized herb among those looking to foster longevity and calm.

Active Compounds and Benefits

Known for its saponins and adaptogenic attributes, Shatavari fortifies the adrenal glands, balances stress-induced hormone production, and offers anti-inflammatory properties that support full-body health. This herb acts gently on the endocrine system, helping to stabilize mood and reinforce emotional resilience while enhancing hydration and soothing tissue.

Most Potent Method of Ingestion

Shatavari is most effective as a powdered supplement mixed into warm milk or as a capsule. Its powder easily blends into herbal tonics or can be added to nourishing drinks for consistent adrenal support. A half teaspoon of Shatavari powder in warm milk daily helps sustain adrenal health. Capsules (500 mg) can be taken once or twice daily for added support.

Simple Recipe: Shatavari Adrenal Tonic

Mix half a teaspoon Shatavari powder into 1 cup warm milk (dairy or plant-based). Add honey for taste. Consume in the evening to nourish adrenal health and calm the nervous system.

Best Herbs to Use Together

Shatavari works harmoniously with ashwagandha for adrenal resilience and complements Gotu Kola for holistic stress support.

ENHANCING MENTAL CLARITY

71. Gotu Kola (Centella asiatica)

Historical Context

Renowned as a sacred herb in Ayurvedic medicine, Gotu Kola has been cherished for its profound impact on cognitive function and memory. This remarkable plant, often called the "herb of longevity," has found its place in traditional Chinese medicine as well, where it has been used to promote mental clarity and emotional balance. Folklore intertwines with its medicinal use, often depicting it as a symbol of wisdom and enlightenment, believed to elevate consciousness and inspire creativity.

Active Compounds and Benefits

Gotu Kola's active compounds, including triterpenes and asiaticoside, significantly enhance blood circulation to the brain and support neuronal health. This herb is celebrated for its ability to reduce anxiety and improve memory, making it a powerful ally for those seeking mental clarity. With its antioxidant properties, Gotu Kola also protects brain cells from oxidative stress, thus promoting overall cognitive vitality.

Most Potent Method of Ingestion

For optimal benefits, Gotu Kola is best consumed as a tincture or in powdered form mixed into smoothies or herbal teas, allowing for quick absorption of its beneficial compounds. A typical tincture dose is 20–30 drops taken two to three times daily. For the powdered form, 1 teaspoon daily is recommended.

Simple Recipe: Gotu Kola Tea

Steep 1 teaspoon of dried Gotu Kola leaves in 1 cup of boiling water for 10–15 minutes. Strain and enjoy, perhaps with a dash of honey for sweetness. This calming tea enhances focus and sharpens the mind.

Best Herbs to Use Together

Combining Gotu Kola with Brahmi amplifies cognitive benefits, fostering a harmonious synergy that promotes mental clarity and emotional stability.

72. Brahmi (*Bacopa monnieri*)

Historical Context

Revered in Ayurvedic tradition, Brahmi has long been a celebrated herb for enhancing intellect and memory. Often linked to divine wisdom, this herb is believed to nurture the mind and spirit, facilitating deeper states of meditation and insight. Its name, derived from "Brahma," the creator in Hindu mythology, signifies its esteemed status in promoting clarity and consciousness, as well as fostering spiritual growth.

Active Compounds and Benefits

Brahmi is rich in bacosides, which support synaptic function and improve the transmission of signals between neurons. This potent herb is known for its ability to enhance cognitive function, boost memory retention, and promote focus while simultaneously reducing anxiety and stress levels. With its neuroprotective properties, Brahmi helps safeguard the brain against age-related decline.

Most Potent Method of Ingestion

Brahmi is best utilized as a tincture or as powdered extract added to food or beverages. Its flavors blend well into herbal smoothies, promoting both taste and health benefits. For cognitive enhancement, 20–30 drops of Brahmi tincture taken twice daily is effective. Alternatively, consuming 300–500 mg of Brahmi powder daily provides supportive benefits.

Simple Recipe: Brahmi Smoothie

Blend 1 banana, 1 cup of spinach, 1 teaspoon of Brahmi powder, and 1 cup of almond milk. Enjoy this nutrient-rich smoothie to boost your focus and nourish your mind.

Best Herbs to Use Together

Brahmi synergizes beautifully with Gotu Kola, enhancing mental clarity and emotional balance.

REDUCING PANIC ATTACKS

73. Blue Vervain (*Verbena hastata*)

Historical Context

Among Native American and European herbalists, blue vervain holds a reputation as a calming and restorative herb. This vibrant plant was often seen as a symbol of divine intervention and protection, used in rituals to ease troubled minds and release emotional blockages. In folklore, it was thought to bring peace to the heart, encouraging resilience and tranquility, especially in times of distress or panic.

Active Compounds and Benefits

Blue vervain is rich in iridoid glycosides, tannins, and essential oils, which contribute to its calming properties. Blue vervain helps relieve physical symptoms of anxiety, such as muscle tightness, headaches, and restlessness. Its nervine properties make it a powerful ally for reducing panic attacks, helping to ease both physical and emotional turmoil.

Most Potent Method of Ingestion

A tincture of blue vervain is especially effective for panic relief due to its rapid absorption and calming impact on the nervous system. Take 20–30 drops of blue vervain tincture up to three times daily, especially during moments of heightened anxiety or before situations that may trigger panic.

Simple Recipe: Blue Vervain Tincture for Calm

Place 1 cup of dried blue vervain leaves in a clean jar and cover with 80-proof vodka. Seal and let sit for 4–6 weeks, shaking gently every few days. Strain and store in a dark bottle. Use during stressful times to reduce panic symptoms.

Best Herbs to Use Together

Blue vervain combines well with corydalis to create a potent remedy for reducing nervous tension and easing panic-related symptoms.

74. Corydalis (*Corydalis yanhusuo*)

Historical Context

Hailing from traditional Chinese medicine, corydalis has been a prized herb for addressing pain and calming the spirit for centuries. Known as "Yan Hu Suo" in Chinese pharmacology, it was historically valued as a remedy for discomfort and anxiety. In folk medicine, corydalis was thought to balance yin and yang energies, promoting inner peace and grounding.

Active Compounds and Benefits

Corydalis contains the powerful alkaloid tetrahydropalmatine (THP), which exerts mild sedative and pain-relieving effects. This compound works by calming the nervous system and reducing physical symptoms associated with anxiety, such as heart palpitations and muscle tension. Due to its soothing properties, corydalis is particularly effective for managing panic attacks.

Most Potent Method of Ingestion

Corydalis is most potent as a capsule or tincture, allowing quick access to its soothing benefits. For panic relief, take 300–400 mg of corydalis in a capsule or 20–30 drops of tincture once or twice daily, ideally at night for calming rest.

Simple Recipe: Corydalis Nighttime Tincture

Place 1 cup of dried corydalis root in a jar, covering it with 80-proof vodka. Seal and store in a cool, dark place for 4–6 weeks, shaking occasionally. Strain and store. Take in the evening to reduce anxiety and encourage restful sleep.

Best Herbs to Use Together

Pairing corydalis with blue vervain enhances both herbs' calming properties, creating a synergy that aids in easing both emotional and physical symptoms of panic.

SUPPORTING LONG-TERM STRESS MANAGEMENT

75. Bay Leaf (*Laurus nobilis*)

Historical Context

Bay leaf has been revered since ancient Greece and Rome as a symbol of wisdom, strength, and resilience. Traditionally used in ritualistic practices to protect against harm, bay leaf was believed to grant mental clarity and emotional strength. Ancient healers often infused this herb into baths or burned it to cleanse both body and spirit. Today, bay leaf continues to be cherished for its soothing properties, particularly in easing chronic stress.

Active Compounds and Benefits

Rich in eugenol, cineole, and myrcene, bay leaf has potent anti-inflammatory, anxiolytic, and soothing properties. These compounds support the body's stress response by relaxing muscle tension and promoting a deep sense of calm. Its gentle effects on the central nervous system make it ideal for long-term stress management.

Most Potent Method of Ingestion

Bay leaf is most effective as a daily infusion or as part of a calming steam inhalation, allowing its essential oils to penetrate deeply into the system. Drink 1–2 cups of bay leaf tea daily to maintain calm and promote resilience against stress.

Simple Recipe: Bay Leaf Calming Infusion

Place 2–3 dried bay leaves in a pot with 2 cups of hot water. Allow to simmer for 10–15 minutes, then strain and cool. Sip slowly, allowing the infusion to relax and soothe the mind.

Best Herbs to Use Together

Bay leaf works harmoniously with velvet bean for comprehensive stress management.

76. Velvet Bean (*Mucuna pruriens*)

Historical Context

Velvet bean has been cherished in Ayurvedic and traditional African medicine as a tonic for mental and physical vitality. In Ayurvedic practices, it is revered as a source of positivity, believed to enhance energy and alleviate low moods. It was known for its uplifting effects and has long been valued as a way to restore balance and promote resilience to long-term stress.

Active Compounds and Benefits

Velvet bean contains high levels of L-dopa, a precursor to dopamine, the "feel-good" neurotransmitter. This compound plays a key role in elevating mood, reducing symptoms of stress, and enhancing focus and motivation. Over time, regular use of velvet bean supports the nervous system's ability to cope with prolonged stress by naturally boosting dopamine levels.

Most Potent Method of Ingestion

Velvet bean works best as a powdered supplement or capsule, providing a sustained release of L-dopa for continuous stress support. Take 300–500 mg of velvet bean powder daily, mixed into warm water or a calming herbal tea, to encourage stress resilience.

Simple Recipe: Mucuna Resilience Powder

Mix a quarter teaspoon of velvet bean powder into a warm, calming tea or blend with a smoothie.

Stir well and sip, allowing the herb to soothe and uplift.

Best Herbs to Use Together

Pairing velvet bean with bay leaf creates a potent combination for long-term stress management, fostering a calm and balanced state over time.

PROMOTING EMOTIONAL WELL-BEING

77. Damiana (*Turnera diffusa*)

Historical Context

Damiana, with its delicate leaves and fragrant flowers, has been cherished since the times of the ancient Maya and Aztec civilizations as a mood-elevating herb. Traditional cultures revered it not only as a tonic for the body but also as an enhancer of emotional well-being and romantic spirit. Historically used in love potions, damiana was believed to awaken joy, support resilience, and inspire a lighthearted connection to life's simple pleasures.

Active Compounds and Benefits

Damiana's magic lies in its blend of flavonoids, terpenoids, and thymol glycosides, which work together to gently lift the mood and calm the mind. These compounds have anxiolytic and mildly euphoric effects, helping to ease feelings of sadness and emotional fatigue.

Most Potent Method of Ingestion

A tincture or mild tea best harnesses damiana's mood-elevating effects, allowing its active compounds to be gradually absorbed. Take 1–2 teaspoons of damiana tincture daily, or enjoy 1–2 cups of tea throughout the day for a sustained mood-lifting effect.

Simple Recipe: Damiana Heart-Lifting Tea

Place 1 tablespoon of dried damiana leaves in a cup. Pour over 8 ounces of hot water and let steep for 10 minutes. Strain and sip slowly.

Best Herbs to Use Together

For enhanced emotional well-being, pair damiana with linden flower to support a peaceful heart and balanced mood.

78. Linden Flower (*Tilia europaea*)

Historical Context

Known as the "tree of love," linden flower has held a special place in European herbal traditions, symbolizing peace and emotional healing. In ancient Germany, the linden tree was a meeting place for communal gatherings and reconciliation, believed to offer comfort to troubled hearts. Linden flower's soothing properties were valued in traditional folk medicine for calming emotional distress and promoting gentle relaxation.

Active Compounds and Benefits

Linden flower contains flavonoids, volatile oils, and mucilage, which provide anti-inflammatory, antispasmodic, and sedative properties.

Most Potent Method of Ingestion

Linden flower is most effective as a tea or gentle herbal infusion, allowing its calming compounds to be absorbed slowly. Enjoy 1–2 cups of linden flower tea daily, particularly in the evening, to promote emotional balance and relaxation.

Simple Recipe: Linden Flower Peaceful Tea

Add 1 tablespoon of dried linden flowers to 1 cup of hot water. Let steep for 10–15 minutes, then strain. Sip warmly, allowing its gentle effects to calm the mind and heart.

Best Herbs to Use Together

Linden flower combines beautifully with damiana, working in harmony to encourage emotional well-being, inner peace, and a sense of stability.

COMBATING FATIGUE

79. Maca (Lepidium meyenii)

Historical Context

Maca, the "Peruvian ginseng," has been cultivated in the high altitudes of the Andes for over 2,000 years. This revered root was cherished by ancient Incan warriors, who believed it gave them stamina and endurance before battles. In its native lands, maca is seen as an adaptogenic gift of resilience, an herb for inner strength, and a natural energy lifter.

Active Compounds and Benefits

Maca's unique alkaloids, glucosinolates, and essential amino acids create a powerful tonic for combating fatigue. It acts on the adrenal glands and endocrine system, helping to balance hormone levels and enhance mental and physical energy. By nourishing the hypothalamus and pituitary, maca also stabilizes the body's response to stress, making it a well-rounded option for battling exhaustion.

Most Potent Method of Ingestion

Maca is most commonly enjoyed as a powder, mixed into smoothies or warm beverages, where it can gradually nourish the body and uplift energy levels. Start with 1–2 teaspoons of maca powder daily, gradually increasing to 1 tablespoon as needed for sustainable energy.

Simple Recipe: Maca Energy Smoothie

Blend 1 teaspoon of maca powder with 1 cup almond milk, a handful of spinach, and half a banana.

Add ice if desired, and blend until smooth. Enjoy as a morning pick-me-up.

Best Herbs to Use Together

For enhanced stamina, pair maca with suma, creating a deeply energizing blend that helps counter physical and mental fatigue.

80. Suma (*Pfaffia paniculata*)

Historical Context
Known as the "Brazilian ginseng," suma root has been prized by Indigenous tribes of the Amazon for its ability to support vitality, strength, and resilience. Suma was traditionally consumed as a fortifying tonic, believed to enhance endurance and foster a grounded energy needed to face the day's challenges.

Active Compounds and Benefits
Suma's rich profile includes saponins, pfaffic acid, and a suite of vitamins and minerals, particularly magnesium and iron. These compounds work synergistically to reduce fatigue, support cellular health, and improve oxygen delivery in the body. As an adaptogen, suma helps regulate the body's stress response, increasing energy reserves without overstimulation and offering a steady, balanced energy boost.

Most Potent Method of Ingestion
Suma is best used in powdered or capsule form, where it can gradually be incorporated into daily routines for steady energy support. Take 1 teaspoon of Suma powder or 500 mg in capsule form once or twice daily, ideally with meals.

Simple Recipe: Suma Energizing Tonic
Stir 1 teaspoon of suma powder into warm water or herbal tea. Add honey if desired. Drink in the morning or early afternoon to support sustained energy.

Best Herbs to Use Together
Combine suma with maca to enhance stamina and resilience, creating a powerful duo for combating fatigue and maintaining steady energy throughout the day.

HERBAL REMEDY VIDEO TUTORIALS BELOW!

Hi there! It's Ava, and I'm thrilled you're exploring my home apothecary book. Are you enjoying the recipes and remedies? I hope they're inspiring you as much as they've rejuvenated me.

Experience Herbalism Like Never Before:

I understand that sometimes reading about processes isn't quite the same as seeing them in action. That's why I've put together an exclusive video playlist just for you! Over the past decade, I've captured my herbalism journey in detail, and these videos are packed with hands-on demonstrations to enhance your learning and skills.

Here is a small portion of what is in the playlist:

bit.ly/homeapothecary2025

- **Respiratory Health:** Learn steam inhalation techniques for sinus congestion and respiratory ailments.
- **Pain and Wound Care:** Discover compresses and salves that soothe muscle pain, reduce inflammation, and heal skin irritations.
- **Digestive Issues:** See how tinctures can aid digestion, boost immunity, and enhance mental clarity.
- **Throat Relief:** Create lozenges for effective relief from sore throats and coughs.
- **Skin Health:** Follow recipes for salves that address cuts, burns, and other skin issues.
- **Overall Wellbeing:** Gain insights into remedies for headaches, sleep disorders, and stress management.
- **And So Much More:** Explore additional herbal practices and remedies that extend even further into holistic health.

Get Started Now!

Prepare your herbal workstation, and explore deeper into the world of herbalism. Scan the QR code or use the link on this page to access the videos. Start your hands-on learning today and bring the power of nature into every aspect of your health.

Happy Healing,

Ava

HERBS FOR
PAIN MANAGEMENT

REDUCING INFLAMMATION

81. Devil's Claw (*Harpagophytum procumbens*)

Historical Context

Originating from the arid landscapes of Southern Africa, Devil's Claw has been treasured for centuries by the Indigenous San and Khoisan peoples. They understood its power to alleviate physical discomfort and swelling, crafting teas and poultices from its dried roots. The herb's name derives from its claw-like fruits.

Active Compounds and Benefits

Devil's Claw is rich in iridoid glycosides, particularly harpagoside, which has shown strong anti-inflammatory and analgesic properties. These compounds work by inhibiting enzymes that promote inflammation, offering relief from swelling and discomfort in joints and tissues. It also supports joint health, making it a sought-after remedy for chronic inflammatory conditions like arthritis and rheumatism. Devil's Claw's potent phytochemicals provide natural relief without the harsh effects of synthetic painkillers.

Most Potent Method of Ingestion

Devil's Claw is most effective as a dried root powder or capsule, taken daily to reduce inflammation gradually. Its benefits build over time. Take 500–1,000 mg of Devil's Claw extract in capsule form twice daily, ideally with meals, to reduce inflammation and ease chronic pain.

Simple Recipe: Devil's Claw Anti-Inflammatory Tea

Simmer 1 teaspoon of Devil's Claw root powder in a cup of water for 10–15 minutes. Strain and drink warm, adding honey if desired, twice a day for best results.

Best Herbs to Use Together

Pair Devil's Claw with turmeric or ginger for a synergistic anti-inflammatory effect. Together, they work to reduce swelling and soothe pain.

82. White Willow Bark (*Salix alba*)

Historical Context

White willow bark has been cherished as a natural remedy for pain and inflammation since ancient times. Used by the Egyptians, Greeks, and Native Americans, this bark became the precursor to modern aspirin due to its powerful pain-relieving properties. Known as nature's painkiller, white willow was often brewed into teas and infusions to reduce fevers and soothe aching joints and muscles.

Active Compounds and Benefits

The bark's main active compound, salicin, converts to salicylic acid in the body, providing anti-inflammatory and analgesic effects. White willow bark also contains polyphenols and flavonoids, which enhance its antioxidant properties, supporting the body in reducing inflammation at a cellular level. Its gentle action is known to relieve chronic pain, inflammation, and joint discomfort without the stomach irritation often associated with synthetic pain relievers.

Most Potent Method of Ingestion

White willow bark is most effective when taken as a decoction or tincture. Capsules or powder form can also be effective for a controlled dose, especially for those sensitive to the taste of the bark. For a decoction, drink one cup a day. Alternatively, take 1–2 ml of tincture, up to three times daily.

Simple Recipe: White Willow Bark Anti-Inflammatory Decoction

Combine 1 teaspoon of white willow bark with 1 cup of water. Simmer gently for 10–15 minutes, then strain. Drink up to two cups daily to help relieve pain and inflammation, especially for conditions like arthritis or muscle soreness.

Best Herbs to Use Together

White willow bark pairs well with turmeric and ginger, both of which have complementary anti-inflammatory effects. Combining with Devil's Claw or meadowsweet can enhance pain relief, while chamomile can add a calming effect.

RELIEVING HEADACHES AND MIGRAINES

83. Feverfew (*Tanacetum parthenium*)

Historical Context

With a name that speaks to its age-old use in "fever-few" remedies, feverfew has been revered across ancient Greek and Roman societies for its soothing properties. Traditionally used to treat inflammation and high fevers, it also earned a reputation as a remedy for persistent headaches and migraines. In folklore, feverfew was known as "the migraine herb," carried by medieval healers as a defense against head pain and ailments related to the nervous system.

Active Compounds and Benefits

The key to feverfew's effectiveness lies in its active compounds, especially parthenolide, a sesquiterpene lactone that plays a critical role in reducing inflammation and constriction of blood vessels, which often trigger migraine headaches. Parthenolide also inhibits serotonin release from blood platelets, reducing tension in head muscles and preventing the onset of headaches. Feverfew's compounds regulate inflammatory pathways and reduce migraines' intensity and frequency, making it a trusted herb for headache prevention.

Most Potent Method of Ingestion

Feverfew works best as a daily supplement in capsule or tincture form for preventive benefits. To prevent migraines, take 150–250 mg of feverfew extract daily, ideally in the morning. Avoid high doses, because excessive intake can cause mouth sores.

Simple Recipe: Feverfew Headache Relief Tincture

Combine 1 part dried feverfew leaves with 4 parts alcohol (vodka works well) in a glass jar. Seal and let sit for 4–6 weeks, shaking every few days. Strain the mixture and store in a dark glass bottle. Take 20–30 drops at the onset of a migraine.

Best Herbs to Use Together

Feverfew pairs well with ginger, which enhances its anti-inflammatory properties and supports digestive comfort, which can be compromised during migraines. Together, they form a potent blend for both preventative care and acute migraine relief.

84. Skullcap (*Scutellaria lateriflora*)

Historical Context

Skullcap has long been revered in traditional Native American medicine for its calming, nerve-soothing properties. Known for promoting relaxation, it was used to ease insomnia, tension, and headaches. Early settlers also cherished the herb as a natural sedative, believed to "comfort the spirit" and reduce ailments linked to mental strain, including migraines and nervous exhaustion.

Active Compounds and Benefits

Skullcap contains flavonoids like baicalin and scutellarin, which are renowned for their anti-inflammatory and anxiolytic properties. These compounds help calm the nervous system, relieve muscle tension, and reduce vascular inflammation—often triggers of tension headaches and migraines. By reducing oxidative stress and inhibiting neurotransmitters that exacerbate pain, skullcap provides a natural solution for pain linked to tension and stress.

Most Potent Method of Ingestion

Skullcap is most effective as an infusion or tincture. Taken as a warm tea, it relaxes both mind and body, while a tincture offers a concentrated form, providing immediate relaxation for nerves and soothing head pain. Take 1–2 drops of skullcap tincture at the first sign of a headache or enjoy a warm cup of skullcap tea as a preventive measure.

Simple Recipe: Skullcap Relaxation Tea

Steep 1–2 teaspoons of dried skullcap leaves in hot water for 10–15 minutes. Strain and drink warm, ideally in the evening or at the onset of headache symptoms. Sweeten with honey if desired.

Best Herbs to Use Together

Combine skullcap with lemon balm for an enhanced calming effect. Together, they create a potent blend that helps relieve stress-related headaches and migraines.

EASING JOINT PAIN AND ARTHRITIS

85. Black Cohosh (*Actaea racemosa*)

Historical Context

Black cohosh, also known as "black snakeroot" or "fairy candle," has been a treasured remedy among Native American tribes and later in Europe for its powerful anti-inflammatory properties. It was originally used to support women's health, relieve menstrual discomfort, and ease labor pains, but it also found its way into remedies for joint pain and arthritis. Its benefits for reducing inflammation and muscle tension became more widely recognized.

Active Compounds and Benefits

The herb's potency for joint pain lies in its active compounds, especially triterpene glycosides and isoferulic acid. These compounds are known for their ability to alleviate inflammation, reduce swelling, and relieve the pain associated with arthritis and rheumatism. Black cohosh also acts as a mild sedative, helping to soothe the nervous system and relieve stress-related muscle pain, a secondary benefit for arthritis sufferers who experience tension alongside joint discomfort.

Most Potent Method of Ingestion

Black cohosh is most effective as a tincture or capsule. A consistent, moderate dose can provide ongoing support for inflammation and chronic joint pain. Take 40–80 mg of black cohosh extract or 1–2 ml of tincture up to three times a day to manage joint pain and reduce inflammation. As a long-term remedy, use periodically to avoid overstimulation.

Simple Recipe: Black Cohosh Anti-Inflammatory Tincture

Place dried black cohosh root in a glass jar and cover with high-proof alcohol (vodka or brandy). Seal the jar and store in a cool, dark place for 4–6 weeks, shaking every few days. Strain and take 1–2 ml up to three times daily to relieve arthritis pain.

Best Herbs to Use Together

Black cohosh combines well with white willow bark, a natural source of salicylates, for enhanced pain relief, providing an all-natural alternative to traditional pain medications for arthritis.

86. Marjoram (*Origanum majorana*)

Historical Context

In Greek and Roman traditions, marjoram was a symbol of happiness and health. It has been used for centuries as a medicinal herb for its warming and soothing properties. Ancient healers cherished this aromatic herb for relieving muscular and joint discomfort.

Active Compounds and Benefits

Rich in carvacrol, rosmarinic acid, and flavonoids, marjoram is a natural anti-inflammatory and antispasmodic. These compounds help to reduce joint inflammation, alleviate stiffness, and support muscle relaxation. Marjoram's warming nature stimulates circulation and offers relief for cold, stiff joints, which makes it useful for those with arthritis in colder climates or during winter months.

Most Potent Method of Ingestion

Marjoram is best applied topically as an infused oil or in a warm compress for targeted joint relief. Its soothing warmth and direct application to painful joints make it an ideal external remedy for arthritis symptoms. Massage a few drops of marjoram-infused oil into sore joints or apply a warm compress made with marjoram tea directly onto painful areas for 10–15 minutes, as needed.

Simple Recipe: Marjoram Joint Relief Oil

Fill a jar with dried marjoram leaves and cover with a carrier oil, such as olive or almond oil. Seal and let infuse in a warm place for 2–3 weeks, shaking occasionally. Strain and massage a few drops of oil into affected joints for soothing relief.

Best Herbs to Use Together

Combine marjoram with ginger to enhance circulation and relieve stiffness, creating a warming, anti-inflammatory remedy for joint pain and arthritis.

ALLEVIATING MUSCLE ACHES

87. Helichrysum (*Helichrysum italicum*)

Historical Context

Revered as the "Immortal Flower," Helichrysum has been cherished in Mediterranean cultures for its healing and anti-inflammatory properties. It was known to the ancient Greeks and became a staple in traditional wounds, inflammation, and muscular pain remedies.

Active Compounds and Benefits

Helichrysum is rich in flavonoids, sesquiterpenes, and acetophenones, all known for their potent anti-inflammatory, analgesic, and regenerative effects. Helichrysum also has powerful antioxidant properties, making it ideal for addressing oxidative stress in overworked muscles.

Most Potent Method of Ingestion

Helichrysum is best used as a topical essential oil or salve for targeted relief. Its compounds readily absorb into the skin, offering rapid relief from inflammation and soreness in strained muscles. Dilute a few drops of Helichrysum essential oil in a carrier oil (such as coconut or olive oil) and massage into sore muscles as needed. Alternatively, use as a compress for deep muscle relief.

Simple Recipe: Helichrysum Muscle Relief Salve

Melt a quarter cup of beeswax and a quarter cup of shea butter over low heat. Stir in 20 drops of Helichrysum essential oil and pour into a small jar. Apply a small amount to sore areas for fast relief.

Best Herbs to Use Together

Pair Helichrysum with arnica for a soothing, anti-inflammatory muscle rub. Together, they provide fast-acting relief for muscular discomfort, whether from exercise, strain, or fatigue.

88. Moringa (*Moringa oleifera*)

Historical Context

Moringa was known as the "Miracle Tree" in Ayurvedic and African traditions and has been valued for its comprehensive medicinal properties. Ancient healers believed its leaves and oils could relieve pain and rejuvenate the body, while also addressing a host of ailments.

Active Compounds and Benefits

Moringa contains isothiocyanates, quercetin, and chlorogenic acid, which work as anti-inflammatory agents to reduce muscle pain and swelling. Additionally, its high concentration of vitamins C and E supports collagen synthesis, aiding in muscular recovery and overall tissue health.

Most Potent Method of Ingestion

Moringa is highly effective in powder or capsule form for internal support, but as an oil, it is perfect for topical applications to sore or tense muscles. Take 1–2 capsules of Moringa daily to promote long-term muscle recovery, or massage a few drops of Moringa oil directly onto affected areas for immediate relief.

Simple Recipe: Moringa Oil Massage Blend

Combine 1 tablespoon of Moringa oil with a few drops of lavender essential oil. Gently massage into sore muscles for soothing relief and relaxation.

Best Herbs to Use Together

Combine Moringa with turmeric to amplify its anti-inflammatory effects, creating a powerful blend that soothes muscles and reduces soreness.

SOOTHING MENSTRUAL CRAMPS

89. Dong Quai (*Angelica sinensis*)

Historical Context

For over a thousand years, this earthy, bittersweet root, known as the "female ginseng," has been used across Asia to balance hormones, strengthen reproductive health, and relieve menstrual discomfort. Ancient healers believed it could increase blood flow and regulate energy, providing natural relief from the painful cramps and emotional fluctuations associated with menstruation.

Active Compounds and Benefits

Dong Quai's medicinal potency lies in its rich blend of coumarins, ferulic acid, and phytosterols, which together work to relax the uterine muscles, reduce inflammation, and improve circulation. Ferulic acid, in particular, is known for its antioxidant and anti-inflammatory properties, helping to ease pain and support overall pelvic health. The phytosterols contribute to hormone balance, making Dong Quai ideal for soothing hormonal discomfort and menstrual cramps.

Most Potent Method of Ingestion

Dong Quai is best utilized as a tincture or decoction for quick absorption and maximum relief from menstrual discomfort. This form allows for a concentrated intake of the herb's active compounds, providing targeted support during menstrual periods. Take 30–40 drops of Dong Quai tincture up to three times daily or brew as a decoction, which can be consumed up to twice daily during the menstrual cycle.

Simple Recipe: Dong Quai Menstrual Relief Decoction

Add 1 teaspoon of dried Dong Quai root to a pot with 1 cup of water. Simmer on low heat for 15 minutes. Strain and drink warm, adding honey if desired.

Best Herbs to Use Together

Dong Quai combines well with black cohosh for enhanced hormone balancing and pain relief.

90. Motherwort (*Leonurus cardiaca*)

Historical Context

Named for its reputation as a "mother's herb," motherwort has been a go-to remedy for women's health concerns since ancient Greece, where it was prescribed to ease childbirth pain and relieve menstrual discomfort. Herbalists chose it for its calming effects on both the mind and body, and it was believed to have a special affinity for the heart and uterus, making it an essential herb for nurturing women's well-being.

Active Compounds and Benefits

Motherwort contains leonurine and stachydrine, alkaloids known for their antispasmodic and relaxant properties, which help relieve uterine cramps and tension. These compounds work synergistically to reduce pain, ease muscle spasms, and calm nervous tension.

Most Potent Method of Ingestion

Motherwort is most effective as a tincture, which provides rapid absorption of its active compounds, particularly during the menstrual period when cramps are most intense. Take 20–30 drops of motherwort tincture up to three times daily as needed to ease menstrual cramps. It can also be used preventatively by beginning a few days before the onset of menstruation.

Simple Recipe: Motherwort Calming Tincture

Place fresh or dried motherwort in a glass jar and cover with high-proof alcohol. Let it sit in a cool, dark place for 4-6 weeks, shaking occasionally. Strain and store in a dropper bottle, taking 20–30 drops as needed for menstrual discomfort.

Best Herbs to Use Together

Motherwort pairs well with cramp bark for a powerful antispasmodic blend that further reduces cramping and tension, offering a holistic approach to menstrual comfort and emotional stability.

SUPPORTING NERVE HEALTH

91. Lion's Mane Mushroom (*Hericium erinaceus*)

Historical Context

With its cascading, white tendrils resembling a lion's mane, this unique mushroom has been honored in East Asian medicine for centuries. Known in Japan as *yamabushitake* and in China as *hou tou gu*, Lion's Mane has traditionally been used to promote cognitive vitality and protect the nervous system. Buddhist monks also used it to enhance mental clarity and focus during meditation. This ancient remedy has recently gained global recognition for its potential in nerve health.

Active Compounds and Benefits

Lion's Mane is celebrated for its neuroprotective compounds—hericenones and erinacines—that support nerve growth and repair. These active ingredients stimulate the production of nerve growth factor (NGF), a protein essential for maintaining, regenerating, and protecting nerve cells. This ability to promote neural health and enhance brain function makes Lion's Mane particularly useful for those seeking to maintain cognitive wellness and protect against neurodegenerative conditions.

Most Potent Method of Ingestion

Lion's Mane is best taken as a dual-extracted tincture or powder for comprehensive nerve support. Take 1-2 teaspoons of Lion's Mane powder daily, mixed into warm water or tea, or 1–2 dropperfuls of a dual-extracted tincture up to twice daily.

Simple Recipe: Lion's Mane Calming Tea

Mix 1 teaspoon of Lion's Mane powder into a cup of warm, non-boiling water. Stir well and add honey for taste if desired. Sip slowly in the evening to unwind and support the nervous system.

Best Herbs to Use Together

Lion's Mane pairs well with ginkgo biloba for enhanced cognitive function.

92. Oat Straw (*Avena sativa*)

Historical Context

In ancient Europe, oat straw was often referred to as "the herb of longevity." Herbalists favored its nourishing properties to relieve exhaustion, soothe nerves, and promote a grounded sense of well-being, particularly for those experiencing anxiety and fatigue.

Active Compounds and Benefits

Oat straw is rich in B vitamins, calcium, and magnesium, all of which are vital for nervous system function. These minerals work synergistically to restore nerve health, alleviate stress, and reduce physical and mental tension. Additionally, its soothing alkaloids and anti-inflammatory properties offer gentle support for rebuilding nerve resilience, making it a valuable herb for those dealing with stress-induced nerve pain.

Most Potent Method of Ingestion

Oat straw is most effective as an infusion, allowing its nutrients to extract fully into hot water. Steep 1 tablespoon of dried oat straw in 1 cup of boiling water for 15–20 minutes, then strain. Drink this infusion 1–2 times daily for calming support.

Simple Recipe: Oat Straw Nerve-Soothing Infusion

Place 1 tablespoon of dried oat straw in a mug and pour 1 cup of boiling water over it. Cover and let steep for 15–20 minutes. Strain and drink, adding honey or lemon, if desired.

Best Herbs to Use Together

Oat Straw combines beautifully with lemon balm, adding additional calming effects, which enhance stress relief and offer gentle nerve support.

TOPICAL PAIN RELIEF

93. Arnica (*Arnica montana*)

Historical Context

Known as the "mountain daisy," arnica has been celebrated for centuries by European herbalists as a potent remedy for bruises, sprains, and muscle injuries. Alpine people traditionally used it for its remarkable ability to reduce swelling and ease pain from physical injuries. This flower, growing high in mountainous regions, became a go-to for reducing soreness after long, strenuous days of work or travel.

Active Compounds and Benefits

Arnica's powerful pain-relieving effects come from compounds like sesquiterpene lactones, flavonoids, and thymol, which work together to reduce inflammation, stimulate circulation, and relieve pain when applied topically. These compounds promote healing in bruised and sore tissues, making arnica ideal for addressing pain caused by muscle strains, minor injuries, and joint inflammation.

Most Potent Method of Ingestion

Arnica is best used externally as a topical salve or gel. Direct application allows the healing compounds to penetrate the skin and target painful areas, offering quick relief. Apply a small amount of arnica salve or gel to the affected area 2–3 times daily, as needed. Do not apply to open wounds or broken skin.

Simple Recipe: Arnica Sore Muscle Salve

Melt a quarter cup of beeswax and a half cup of olive oil in a double boiler. Add 2 tablespoons of dried arnica flowers and let infuse on low heat for 1–2 hours. Strain, pour into a jar, and let cool. Apply a small amount to sore muscles or joints.

Best Herbs to Use Together

Arnica pairs well with comfrey for enhanced healing of bruises and muscle pain, offering a complementary mix that promotes faster recovery from minor injuries.

94. Tamanu Oil (*Calophyllum inophyllum*)

Historical Context

Indigenous to Southeast Asia and Polynesia, Tamanu oil has been revered as a sacred healer by island cultures. It was known as "beauty leaf oil," and this rich green oil was traditionally applied to burns, wounds, and skin inflammations. It was often seen as a gift of healing from the gods.

Active Compounds and Benefits

Tamanu oil contains calophyllolide and inophyllum, compounds known for their anti-inflammatory and analgesic properties. These compounds are especially effective in reducing pain and swelling while promoting skin regeneration. Tamanu oil's high content of fatty acids and antioxidants makes it ideal for soothing sore joints, burns, and injuries, reducing pain through deep, moisturizing relief.

Most Potent Method of Ingestion

Tamanu oil works best applied directly to affected areas. This allows it to penetrate the skin deeply and provide extended relief for pain and inflammation. Apply a few drops of Tamanu oil to the painful area 2–3 times daily, massaging gently into the skin.

Simple Recipe: Tamanu Healing Balm

Mix a half cup of Tamanu oil with a quarter cup of shea butter, and melt in a double boiler. Once melted, pour into a small jar and let cool. Use a small amount on sore or inflamed areas for soothing relief.

Best Herbs to Use Together

Tamanu oil works synergistically with St. John's Wort oil, providing a dual-action approach to reduce pain and inflammation.

MANAGING CHRONIC PAIN

95. Rehmannia (*Rehmannia glutinosa*)

Historical Context

In traditional Chinese medicine (TCM), Rehmannia, or *di huang*, has long been treasured for its ability to nurture vitality and alleviate chronic discomfort. It was known as a "blood tonic" in TCM, and this root has been used to soothe conditions such as arthritis and persistent pain. Its grounding properties are believed to balance the body's energies.

Active Compounds and Benefits

Rehmannia's healing power comes from iridoid glycosides, particularly catalpol, which is renowned for its anti-inflammatory and immune-modulating effects. These compounds work together to ease chronic inflammation and support adrenal function. This makes Rehmannia particularly valuable for those experiencing pain tied to adrenal fatigue or immune-related conditions. Its adaptogenic qualities help the body handle stress, addressing the roots of chronic pain.

Most Potent Method of Ingestion

Rehmannia is most effective as a decoction or in powdered form. Decoctions allow the compounds to concentrate, providing more sustained pain relief and calming effects when taken regularly. Drink 1–2 cups decoction daily, adjusting based on tolerance.

Simple Recipe: Rehmannia Anti-Inflammatory Decoction

Combine 1–2 teaspoons of dried Rehmannia root with 1 cup water in a pot. Simmer on low heat for 20–30 minutes. Strain and drink once cooled. Take once or twice daily to help manage chronic pain and inflammation.

Best Herbs to Use Together

Rehmannia combines well with astragalus for immune support and anti-inflammatory benefits, creating a powerful duo to help relieve chronic pain from autoimmune conditions.

96. Sarsaparilla (*Smilax ornata*)

Historical Context

Sarsaparilla was traditionally used by Indigenous tribes in America and Asia as a blood purifier and pain reliever. Known for its grounding, earthy qualities, it was often employed to treat joint pain, inflammation, and skin conditions. Spanish explorers later brought sarsaparilla to Europe, where it became popular as a tonic for vitality and relief from chronic ailments.

Active Compounds and Benefits

Sarsaparilla contains saponins, which have anti-inflammatory and detoxifying properties, as well as plant sterols that support hormonal balance. These compounds work together to alleviate pain, reduce swelling, and enhance detoxification, offering relief for chronic pain linked to inflammation and toxicity. Sarsaparilla's effectiveness in managing joint pain makes it an enduring favorite among those seeking natural pain relief.

Most Potent Method of Ingestion

Sarsaparilla is most beneficial as a tea or tincture, which allows for efficient absorption and regular, low-dose intake to support gradual pain reduction and detoxification.

Simple Recipe: Sarsaparilla Pain Relief Tea

Add 1–2 teaspoons of dried sarsaparilla root to a cup of hot water. Steep for 10–15 minutes, strain, and drink. Enjoy once or twice daily for pain relief.

Best Herbs to Use Together

Sarsaparilla pairs well with burdock root for enhanced detoxifying effects, making this duo effective for those seeking relief from chronic pain linked to inflammation and toxin buildup in the body. Together, they provide a cleansing, soothing remedy for persistent discomfort.

REDUCING PAIN FROM INJURIES

97. Yarrow (*Achillea millefolium*)

Historical Context

Yarrow is known as "warrior's herb" or "soldier's woundwort" and has been revered for centuries as a remedy for pain and wound healing. Its use dates back to ancient Greece, where Achilles employed it to treat soldiers' injuries on the battlefield, inspiring its Latin name, *Achillea*. Yarrow has maintained its reputation in folk medicine as an essential herb for soothing pain, stopping bleeding, and aiding in wound recovery.

Active Compounds and Benefits

Yarrow's power lies in its array of flavonoids, tannins, and alkaloids, which exhibit anti-inflammatory and analgesic effects. These compounds help reduce swelling and promote healing, making yarrow particularly effective for cuts, bruises, and injuries with inflammation. Its antispasmodic properties further ease muscle tension around wounds, creating a holistic approach to pain relief and injury care.

Most Potent Method of Ingestion

Yarrow works best as a poultice or infused oil applied directly to the affected area, where its compounds can swiftly relieve pain, reduce inflammation, and accelerate the healing process.

Simple Recipe: Yarrow Healing Poultice

Crush fresh yarrow leaves and flowers to release their juices. Apply the crushed plant matter directly onto the affected area. Secure with a cloth or gauze, leaving it in place for 15–20 minutes. Repeat as necessary to reduce pain and swelling.

Best Herbs to Use Together

Yarrow pairs well with comfrey for enhanced tissue repair and arnica to alleviate pain and bruising.

98. Blue Lotus (*Nymphaea caerulea*)

Historical Context

The blue lotus flower was sacred in ancient Egyptian culture, and celebrated as a symbol of rebirth, tranquility, and relief. Traditionally, it was used as a soothing remedy to ease pain and induce relaxation, often employed in poultices or as a steeped flower infusion for injury and muscular discomfort. The blue lotus was believed to elevate spirits and aid in the gentle relief of both physical and emotional distress.

Active Compounds and Benefits

Blue lotus is rich in alkaloids, notably aporphine, which delivers mild sedative effects, promoting relaxation and natural pain relief. Its mild euphoria-inducing qualities make it especially useful for easing the discomfort and tension often associated with injuries. Blue lotus also has natural antispasmodic properties, which help to reduce muscle contractions around injured areas.

Most Potent Method of Ingestion

Blue Lotus is most effective as a topical oil or infused salve for injury-related pain relief. Use a few drops of blue lotus–infused oil on the affected area, gently massaging into the skin to relieve pain and tension. Repeat as needed for continued relief.

Simple Recipe: Blue Lotus Pain Relief Oil

Steep dried blue lotus flowers in a carrier oil, such as jojoba or almond, for 2–3 weeks in a warm, dark place. Strain the oil and store it in a glass bottle. Apply a few drops to the affected area, massaging gently to relieve pain and calm the nerves.

Best Herbs to Use Together

Blue lotus blends beautifully with lavender and chamomile for a calming, anti-inflammatory effect. This combination is especially soothing for those recovering from injury, offering both physical relief and gentle emotional support as the body heals.

NATURAL ALTERNATIVES TO PAINKILLERS

99. Magnolia Bark (*Magnolia officinalis*)

Historical Context

Traditional Chinese medicine used magnolia bark for centuries to treat pain, anxiety, and inflammation. It was known as *houpu* in Chinese herbalism and was often given as a remedy for tension, digestive distress, and inflammatory conditions. For its calming yet potent effects, magnolia bark has gradually become popular worldwide as a gentle, natural alternative to painkillers.

Active Compounds and Benefits

The primary active compounds in magnolia bark are honokiol and magnolol, which possess anti-inflammatory, antispasmodic, and analgesic properties. These compounds work by modulating the body's inflammatory response and inhibiting pain pathways, offering relief without harsh side effects. Magnolia bark also has a mild sedative effect, helping to ease tension-related pain while promoting a sense of calm.

Most Potent Method of Ingestion

Magnolia bark is most effective when used as a tincture or capsule. These forms allow for concentrated doses of the herb's active compounds, offering quick and potent pain relief. Take 200–400 mg of magnolia bark extract or 1–2 ml of tincture up to three times daily for pain relief. Start with a lower dose to assess tolerance and gradually increase if needed.

Simple Recipe: Magnolia Bark Tincture

Place dried magnolia bark in a glass jar and cover with high-proof alcohol (vodka or brandy). Seal the jar and store it in a cool, dark place for 4–6 weeks, shaking every few days. Strain and take 1–2 ml up to three times daily to ease pain and reduce inflammation.

Best Herbs to Use Together

Combine magnolia bark with skullcap for enhanced pain-relieving effects and added relaxation. This duo is particularly useful for those dealing with stress-related pain.

100. Hops (*Humulus lupulus*)

Historical Context

Hops were historically valued in Europe and North America and were first popularized as a key ingredient in beer brewing. However, their medicinal properties for calming the nervous system and reducing pain quickly gained recognition, making hops an essential part of herbal pain remedies. Known for their sedative and anti-inflammatory qualities, hops have been used to ease pain, promote relaxation, and relieve muscle tension for centuries.

Active Compounds and Benefits

Hops contain bitter acids, such as humulone and lupulone, which are known for their anti-inflammatory and analgesic effects. These compounds target inflammatory pain, particularly in cases of arthritis or muscle pain. Hops also contain the essential oils myrcene and humulene, which have calming, antispasmodic effects and can reduce pain caused by muscle contractions or tension.

Most Potent Method of Ingestion

Hops are best consumed as a tincture or in capsule form for effective pain relief, particularly for inflammatory pain. Take 200–400 mg of hops extract or 1–2 ml of tincture up to three times a day. Alternatively, a warm compress made from hops can be applied externally for direct relief of muscle tension or localized pain. Apply the hops warm compress to the affected area for 10–15 minutes.

Simple Recipe: Hops Pain Relief Compress

Place 1–2 tablespoons of dried hops flowers in a bowl and cover with hot water. Allow it to steep for 5–10 minutes, then strain. Soak a cloth in the infusion, wring out the excess, and apply to the affected area for 10–15 minutes.

Best Herbs to Use Together

Hops pair well with valerian root for pain relief and deep relaxation. This mix is especially beneficial for individuals experiencing pain alongside insomnia or anxiety.

HERBS FOR
IMMUNE SUPPORT

BOOSTING OVERALL IMMUNITY

101. Cayenne (*Capsicum annuum*)

Historical Context

Long cherished in traditional medicine across the Americas and Asia, cayenne pepper has been a powerful ally for boosting circulation and overall vitality. Its vibrant red hue has symbolized its heat and potency for centuries, particularly in Ayurvedic and Native American practices, where it was used to stimulate digestion and invigorate the body. This herb was known for its warming energy and has more recently been recognized as a natural immune booster, enhancing the body's defenses.

Active Compounds and Benefits

The primary active compound, capsaicin, is responsible for cayenne's fiery kick and many of its health benefits. Capsaicin is known to stimulate circulation, which can help the immune system function more efficiently by ensuring a rapid transport of immune cells. Cayenne is rich in vitamins C, B6, and A, along with essential minerals, and supports immune resilience, fortifying the body against seasonal illnesses. Its antioxidant properties also reduce oxidative stress, aiding in the prevention of cellular damage.

Most Potent Method of Ingestion

Cayenne works well in powder or capsule form for convenient dosing, but a warm infusion can be particularly effective during immune challenges, because it allows the capsaicin to deliver its full warming, circulatory benefits throughout the body. For an immune-supporting tonic, drink 1 cup (8 ounces) every day. For capsules, follow the recommended dosage on the product, often around 500 mg once or twice daily.

Simple Recipe: Cayenne Immune Tonic

Mix a pinch of Cayenne powder, the juice of half a lemon, and a teaspoon of honey in 8 ounces of warm water. Stir well and sip slowly to boost circulation and immune response, especially at the onset of cold symptoms.

Best Herbs to Use Together

Combine cayenne with ginger and garlic for a potent immune blend, since these herbs share warming and antibacterial properties. It also pairs well with echinacea and elderberry for comprehensive immune support.

102. Siberian Ginseng (*Eleutherococcus senticosus*)

Historical Context

Known as a "tonic for all seasons" in traditional Chinese medicine, Siberian Ginseng, or *Eleuthero*, has long been revered for its adaptogenic and immune-supportive properties. It was used by Russian athletes and cosmonauts for its stamina-enhancing effects and has a reputation for boosting vitality, endurance, and overall resilience, which makes it an ideal herb for enhancing immune function.

Active Compounds and Benefits

Siberian Ginseng contains eleutherosides, a group of compounds that enhance the immune response. These compounds help the body adapt to physical and mental stress, making it less susceptible to illness. The herb also improves the activity of immune cells, such as natural killer cells and macrophages, which are crucial for defending the body against infections.

Most Potent Method of Ingestion

Siberian Ginseng is best taken as a tincture or capsule for sustained immune support. This adaptogen can be incorporated into daily routines to build resilience, particularly during high-stress periods or colder months. Take 300–400 mg of Siberian Ginseng extract or 1–2 ml of tincture once or twice daily. Consistent use over time is recommended for maximum benefits.

Simple Recipe: Siberian Ginseng Vitality Tincture

Place dried Siberian Ginseng root in a glass jar and cover with high-proof alcohol. Seal the jar and let sit for 6-8 weeks in a cool, dark place, shaking occasionally. Strain and take 1–2 ml daily to support immunity and energy.

Best Herbs to Use Together

Pair Siberian Ginseng with astragalus for enhanced immune and adaptogenic effects. Together, they provide a balanced approach to fortifying the body's defenses year-round.

PREVENTING COLDS AND FLU

103. Hyssop (*Hyssopus officinalis*)

Historical Context

Hyssop has been revered since ancient times and is a sacred herb in Greek, Roman, and Hebrew traditions. Its aromatic, cleansing properties make it popular for warding off infections and purifying spaces. Herbalists use hyssop to soothe respiratory ailments and prevent seasonal illnesses.

Active Compounds and Benefits

Hyssop's potency lies in its volatile oils, such as pinocamphone and thujone, along with flavonoids and tannins. These compounds work together to relieve respiratory congestion, reduce inflammation, and combat infection-causing microbes. Its antiviral and expectorant properties make it highly effective in preventing colds and flu.

Most Potent Method of Ingestion

Hyssop is best enjoyed as a tea or steam inhalation to maximize its respiratory benefits. The heat helps release its essential oils, offering direct relief to the respiratory system. As a preventive, hyssop tea can be sipped regularly during colder months or flu season to fortify the body's defenses. Drink 1 cup of hyssop tea up to three times daily as a preventive measure. For steam inhalation, add a handful of dried hyssop to a bowl of hot water, cover your head with a towel, and inhale deeply for 5–10 minutes.

Simple Recipe: Hyssop Immune-Boosting Tea

Steep 1 teaspoon of dried hyssop leaves in 1 cup of boiling water for 10 minutes. Strain and enjoy up to three times daily during cold and flu season.

Best Herbs to Use Together

Pair hyssop with thyme for added antimicrobial and respiratory support. Together, they create a powerful defense against respiratory pathogens and seasonal infections.

104. Sage (*Salvia officinalis*)

Historical Context

Sage has been cherished across cultures as a symbol of wisdom, protection, and healing. Ancient herbalists prized it for its ability to enhance longevity and preserve health, often using it in remedies to prevent infection and boost immunity. Its name, derived from the Latin *salvere*, meaning "to heal," speaks to its long-standing role in protecting the body from illness.

Active Compounds and Benefits

Sage contains rosmarinic acid, camphor, and flavonoids, which possess powerful antimicrobial, antioxidant, and anti-inflammatory properties. These compounds strengthen the immune system and protect against the common cold and flu by reducing inflammation and neutralizing harmful pathogens.

Most Potent Method of Ingestion

Sage is highly effective as a tea or gargle, allowing its antibacterial and antiviral properties to target the throat and respiratory tract directly. Drink 1 cup of sage tea up to twice daily as a preventive measure, or use as a gargle to relieve throat discomfort.

Simple Recipe: Sage Throat-Soothing Gargle

Steep 1 tablespoon of dried sage leaves in 1 cup of hot water for 15 minutes. Let cool, then gargle for 30 seconds to soothe sore throats and kill pathogens.

Best Herbs to Use Together

Sage combines well with echinacea for a synergistic immune boost. Together, these herbs create a powerful tonic to defend against colds and flu, with sage providing antimicrobial action and echinacea strengthening immune response.

SUPPORTING RECOVERY FROM ILLNESS

105. Fenugreek (*Trigonella foenum-graecum*)

Historical Context

Fenugreek, revered as both a culinary spice and medicinal herb, has a rich history in Ayurvedic and Middle Eastern medicine for its ability to nourish and restore. It was known as a restorative tonic and was commonly used in traditional medicine to support those recovering from illness, aiding in rebuilding strength and improving digestive health.

Active Compounds and Benefits

Fenugreek is abundant in saponins, alkaloids, and vitamins A, B, and C, which play crucial roles in immune support and recovery. Its high mucilage content soothes the digestive tract, reduces inflammation, and encourages appetite—a vital factor in regaining strength after illness. The herb's antioxidant properties help to neutralize free radicals in the body, supporting cellular repair and overall rejuvenation.

Most Potent Method of Ingestion

Fenugreek seeds are best consumed as an infusion or decoction to extract their soothing and restorative qualities. For digestive support, fenugreek poultices can also provide relief from bloating or stomach discomfort, which is often common during recovery. Drink 1 cup of fenugreek decoction daily during the recovery phase. For a poultice, mix ground seeds with warm water and apply to the stomach area for 15–20 minutes to relieve digestive discomfort.

Simple Recipe: Fenugreek Restorative Decoction

Boil 1 tablespoon of fenugreek seeds in 2 cups of water for 10–15 minutes. Strain and sip slowly, especially after meals, to aid digestion and encourage a gentle return to strength.

Best Herbs to Use Together

Combine fenugreek with licorice root for additional soothing properties, creating a powerful duo that supports digestion, reduces inflammation, and provides a gentle boost to the immune system.

106. Andrographis (*Andrographis paniculata*)

Historical Context

Andrographis, often called the "King of Bitters," is a popular herb in traditional Chinese and Ayurvedic medicine for its powerful immune-supporting and anti-inflammatory properties. Historically, it was used to clear heat and relieve infections, making it a go-to remedy for those recovering from fever and illness, particularly respiratory infections.

Active Compounds and Benefits

This herb is rich in andrographolides, bitter compounds known for their potent immune-enhancing effects. Andrographis supports faster recovery by stimulating immune response, reducing inflammation, and promoting detoxification. Its antiviral and antibacterial qualities also help prevent secondary infections.

Most Potent Method of Ingestion

Andrographis is most potent in capsule or powder form to ensure consistent dosage, especially during recovery. For respiratory relief, an herbal steam using Andrographis leaves or powder can help soothe the airways and clear congestion, supporting respiratory health in the recovery phase. Take 400–600 mg of Andrographis extract up to twice daily to support immunity.

Simple Recipe: Andrographis Immune-Boosting Steam

Add 1 teaspoon of Andrographis powder to a bowl of steaming hot water. Cover your head with a towel, lean over the bowl, and inhale deeply for 5–10 minutes to relieve congestion and boost recovery.

Best Herbs to Use Together

Pair Andrographis with astragalus to enhance immune resilience. Together, these herbs give a gentle boost to energy and endurance.

ANTIVIRAL SUPPORT

107. Neem (*Azadirachta indica*)

Historical Context

Neem, known as "Nature's Pharmacy" in Ayurveda, has been cherished in India for thousands of years for its extensive medicinal properties. Traditionally, neem leaves, bark, and oil were used to combat infections, purify the blood, and protect against viral and bacterial pathogens. Its role as a powerful antiviral agent earned it a sacred place in homes, where its branches were even hung at doorways to ward off illnesses.

Active Compounds and Benefits

Neem is rich in antiviral compounds, including nimbin, quercetin, and azadirachtin, each of which contributes to its effectiveness in fighting infections. These active constituents help disrupt viral replication, strengthen immune response, and offer anti-inflammatory benefits. Neem's purifying properties also support the liver and detoxification processes.

Most Potent Method of Ingestion

Neem is commonly ingested as a capsule or tincture for consistent antiviral support. Externally, neem oil or a poultice can be applied to the skin to protect against infections or soothe irritated areas. Due to its potency, neem should be taken periodically rather than continuously. Take 1–2 neem capsules daily or 1 ml of tincture once a day for a week. For topical application, mix a few drops of neem oil with a carrier oil and apply as needed for skin support.

Simple Recipe: Neem Antiviral Tincture

Place dried neem leaves or powder in a glass jar and cover with alcohol, such as vodka. Seal and store in a cool, dark place for 4–6 weeks, shaking occasionally. Strain and take 1 ml as needed, or apply diluted for skin relief.

Best Herbs to Use Together

Combine neem with turmeric for enhanced antiviral effects.

108. Elderflower (*from Sambucus nigra*)

Historical Context

Elderflower, the delicate blossom of the elder tree, has been a staple in European folk medicine for centuries. It was known for its antiviral and immune-boosting qualities and was traditionally used in teas and tonics. Elderflower was believed to purify the blood and combat colds, flus, and other respiratory ailments.

Active Compounds and Benefits

Rich in flavonoids, chlorogenic acid, and essential oils, elderflower possesses antiviral, anti-inflammatory, and antioxidant properties. These compounds help prevent viral replication, reduce fever, and support respiratory health. Elderflower is particularly effective for soothing the mucous membranes and aiding in the recovery of common colds, sinusitis, and flu symptoms.

Most Potent Method of Ingestion

Elderflower is most commonly prepared as a tea or syrup for respiratory and immune support. It can also be used in a steam inhalation to clear congestion and relieve nasal passages during viral infections. For tea, steep 1–2 teaspoons of dried elderflower in a cup of hot water for 10 minutes, then strain. Drink up to three times daily during cold or flu season for added antiviral support.

Simple Recipe: Elderflower Immune-Boosting Syrup

Combine 1 cup of dried elderflowers with 2 cups of water and simmer for 20 minutes. Strain, mix with honey, and take 1 tablespoon as needed during illness.

Best Herbs to Use Together

Elderflower pairs well with echinacea to enhance immune resilience, creating a potent, antiviral combination that supports faster recovery and helps protect against seasonal illnesses.

STRENGTHENING RESPIRATORY IMMUNITY

109. Osha Root (*Ligusticum porteri*)

Historical Context

Osha root, revered by Indigenous peoples of the Rocky Mountains and Southwestern United States, is known as a powerful ally for respiratory health. For centuries, it was used by Native American tribes as a remedy for colds, coughs, and respiratory infections, believed to provide deep support to the lungs and bronchial system. Osha was traditionally chewed or brewed into a tea to ease breathing difficulties, a practice passed down through generations.

Active Compounds and Benefits

The potent compounds in osha, including ligustilide and other aromatic oils, offer strong antimicrobial, anti-inflammatory, and expectorant properties. These active ingredients stimulate circulation in the respiratory system, helping to break up mucus and clear congestion, while soothing irritated tissues. Osha root is particularly effective in relieving symptoms of bronchitis, asthma, and chronic coughs.

Most Potent Method of Ingestion

Osha root is most commonly used as a tincture or decoction. The root can also be chewed or brewed into a tea for a milder, more gradual effect, particularly for those suffering from chronic respiratory issues. For tincture use, take 1–2 ml up to three times daily. As a tea, steep 1 teaspoon of dried osha root in hot water for 10–15 minutes, then strain and drink up to twice daily for respiratory support.

Simple Recipe: Osha Root Respiratory Tincture

Place dried osha root in a jar and cover with high-proof alcohol (vodka or brandy). Seal and store in a cool, dark place for 4–6 weeks, shaking occasionally. Strain and take 1–2 ml as needed to ease congestion and boost respiratory immunity.

Best Herbs to Use Together

Combine osha with echinacea for a potent respiratory tonic. This creates a dual-action remedy that strengthens both the immune and respiratory systems simultaneously.

110. Coltsfoot (*Tussilago farfara*)

Historical Context

Coltsfoot, a plant named for its hoof-shaped leaves, has a long history of use in Europe and Asia for treating respiratory ailments. It was traditionally a gentle yet effective remedy for coughs, asthma, and other lung-related issues. Herbalists commonly used coltsfoot in syrup and lozenge forms to ease respiratory distress and strengthen lung health.

Active Compounds and Benefits

Coltsfoot contains mucilage, flavonoids, and tannins, which provide therapeutic effects. The mucilage soothes and coats irritated throat tissues, while the flavonoids offer anti-inflammatory and antioxidant properties that help to strengthen the immune system and combat respiratory infections. Coltsfoot acts as an expectorant, helping to loosen mucus and clear the airways, making it ideal for chronic coughs, bronchitis, and asthma.

Most Potent Method of Ingestion

Coltsfoot is best used as a tea, syrup, or lozenge to soothe and clear the respiratory system. Its gentle, calming effects make it suitable for acute and chronic respiratory conditions, offering relief without harsh side effects. For tea, steep 1–2 teaspoons of dried coltsfoot leaves in hot water for 10–15 minutes and strain. Drink up to three times a day to support respiratory immunity and ease coughs.

Simple Recipe: Coltsfoot Soothing Syrup

Simmer 1 cup of dried coltsfoot leaves in 2 cups of water for 20 minutes. Strain, mix with honey or glycerin and store in a bottle. Take 1 tablespoon as needed for coughs and respiratory support.

Best Herbs to Use Together

Combine coltsfoot with licorice root for a powerful, soothing duo. Licorice enhances the expectorant properties of coltsfoot while also providing additional immune support.

HERBS FOR IMMUNE SUPPORT

BALANCING THE IMMUNE RESPONSE

111. Red Clover (*Trifolium pratense*)

Historical Context

Red clover, known for its vibrant pink blossoms, has a rich history of use in Europe, Asia, and North America. It's a gentle yet potent herb employed for centuries as a detoxifying and immune-supportive remedy. In traditional European herbal medicine, red clover was used to promote overall health, balance the body, and support the blood.

Active Compounds and Benefits

Red clover contains isoflavones, flavonoids, and coumarins, all of which support immune system balance. The isoflavones, in particular, are thought to have adaptogenic properties, helping to regulate the body's immune response to both acute and chronic stressors. Red clover also acts as a mild lymphatic stimulant, helping to clear toxins from the body and improve circulation. It is often used to promote a healthy inflammatory response and improve the body's ability to fight off infections.

Most Potent Method of Ingestion

Red clover is best consumed as an infusion or in capsule form, allowing the active compounds to be absorbed into the bloodstream gradually. The infusion offers a soothing way to support the body's immune system. For infusion, drink 1–2 cups daily for overall immune support. For capsules, follow the manufacturer's recommendations, typically 500 mg once or twice daily.

Simple Recipe: Red Clover Immune-Boosting Infusion

Place 1–2 teaspoons of dried red clover flowers into a teapot or cup. Pour hot water over the flowers, cover, and steep for 10–15 minutes. Strain and enjoy as a daily tonic to support balanced immune function.

Best Herbs to Use Together

Red clover pairs beautifully with echinacea for an enhanced immune boost. While red clover works to balance and detoxify the system, echinacea strengthens the immune system's response to infection.

112. Blessed Thistle (*Cnicus benedictus*)

Historical Context

Blessed thistle, with its striking thistle-like flowers, has been a prominent herb in European and traditional Mediterranean medicine for centuries. It is known for its bitter taste and has been used to stimulate digestion, improve liver health, and support the immune system. Historically, it was considered a "blessing" for its ability to invigorate the body.

Active Compounds and Benefits

Blessed thistle contains cnicin, a bitter compound that stimulates the immune system and promotes the production of bile, aiding detoxification. It is also rich in flavonoids, which have antioxidant properties that help reduce oxidative stress and support healthy immune function. This herb is particularly useful for balancing the body's inflammatory responses, improving digestion, and providing immune support.

Most Potent Method of Ingestion

Blessed thistle is most effective as a tincture, infusion, or capsule. The tincture allows for a concentrated, quick-acting dose that can provide immediate support to the immune system. The infusion offers a gentler approach, perfect for those who wish to include the herb in their daily routine without the intense bitterness of the raw plant. For tincture, take 1–2 ml up to three times daily. For infusion, drink up to twice a day. For capsules, follow the dosage instructions on the product label.

Simple Recipe: Blessed Thistle Immune-Boosting Infusion

Add 1 teaspoon of dried blessed thistle herb to a cup of hot water. Steep for 10–15 minutes, then strain. Drink once or twice daily to promote immune health and improve digestion.

Best Herbs to Use Together

Pair blessed thistle with goldenseal for a powerful immune-boosting combination. Goldenseal's antimicrobial and immune-stimulating properties complement the detoxifying and digestive-supportive benefits of blessed thistle, creating a comprehensive remedy for balancing the immune system.

SUPPORTING GUT-ASSOCIATED LYMPHOID TISSUE (GALT)

113. Fennel (*Foeniculum vulgare*)

Historical Context

Fennel is a fragrant herb with feathery fronds and a sweet, anise-like flavor. This herb has been used in culinary and medicinal traditions for thousands of years. It was highly valued in ancient Greek, Roman, and Egyptian cultures for its digestive benefits and ability to support overall health. Fennel's connection to gut health goes beyond its ability to ease indigestion; it has long been considered a remedy for maintaining the balance of the gut-associated lymphoid tissue (GALT), an essential part of the body's immune system that resides in the gut.

Active Compounds and Benefits

Fennel is rich in antioxidants, particularly flavonoids and phenolic compounds, which help protect the body from oxidative stress. The volatile oils in fennel, such as anethole, fenchone, and estragole, are responsible for their anti-inflammatory and carminative properties, making them highly effective in soothing the digestive tract. Fennel's ability to regulate gut flora and improve digestive health supports the proper functioning of the GALT. It also helps regulate intestinal motility, enhancing nutrient absorption.

Most Potent Method of Ingestion

Fennel is most effective when taken as an infusion, tincture, or in powder form. The infusion is gentle on the digestive system, allowing the body to absorb the herb's nutrients while promoting optimal gut function. Fennel seeds can also be chewed directly after meals to aid digestion. Drink 2–3 cups of fennel infusion daily to support gut health. As a tincture, take 1–2 ml three times daily.

Simple Recipe: Fennel Digestive Tonic

Place 1–2 teaspoons of fennel seeds in a cup. Pour hot water over the seeds and steep for 10 minutes. Strain and drink to promote digestive and immune health, supporting GALT function.

Best Herbs to Use Together

Combine fennel with marshmallow root for a soothing, anti-inflammatory digestive blend. While fennel regulates gut health and supports GALT, marshmallow root offers gentle mucilage that protects the digestive lining and supports immune function.

114. Chicory Root (*Cichorium intybus*)

Historical Context

Chicory is a hardy herb with blue flowers that has a long history in European folk medicine. For centuries, has been used to support liver and digestive health. Its bitter taste made it a traditional remedy to enhan digestion, stimulate bile production, and improve the function of the gut-associated lymphoid tissue (GALT In medieval times, chicory was prized for its ability to purify blood and promote overall vitality, making it essential herb in supporting the body's natural defenses.

Active Compounds and Benefits

Chicory root contains inulin, a prebiotic fiber that supports healthy gut bacteria and helps balance t microbiome. This prebiotic effect is key for maintaining GALT, which is directly influenced by gut flo health. Chicory also contains sesquiterpene lactones, which have anti-inflammatory properties and may he modulate immune responses. The bitters in the chicory stimulate bile production, aiding in digestion a nutrient absorption.

Most Potent Method of Ingestion

Chicory root is most effective when taken as a decoction or in powdered form. The decoction extracts t bitter compounds that stimulate digestion and support gut function, making it an ideal remedy for improvi GALT health. Chicory root is also available as a coffee substitute, which can be enjoyed regularly for digestive benefits. For a decoction, drink once or twice daily to support digestion and gut health. As powdered supplement, take 1–2 teaspoons mixed into water or smoothies.

Simple Recipe: Chicory Root Digestive Decoction

Place 1–2 teaspoons of dried chicory root in a pot with 1 cup of water. Simmer for 10–15 minutes, then strai Drink once or twice a day to improve digestion and support GALT health.

Best Herbs to Use Together

Combine chicory with dandelion root for a powerful digestive and immune-boosting combination. Whi chicory stimulates bile production and supports gut flora, dandelion enhances detoxification and improv liver health.

DETOXIFYING THE BODY

115. Red Root (*Ceanothus americanus*)

Historical Context

Known as "New Jersey tea," Red Root has a long history in traditional Native American medicine. Indigenous tribes valued it for its detoxifying properties, particularly for supporting lymphatic health and aiding in the removal of toxins from the body. In the 18th century, Red Root gained attention from European settlers for its effectiveness in treating congested lymph and supporting the body's natural detoxification processes, earning its reputation as a "blood purifier" and detoxifier.

Active Compounds and Benefits

Red Root contains potent alkaloids, flavonoids, and tannins, which work synergistically to promote detoxification, improve circulation, and support the lymphatic system. The herb stimulates lymph flow, helping to clear toxins from the tissues and reduce swelling or inflammation associated with toxin buildup. Red Root also has mild diuretic properties, further aiding the body in flushing out waste products. Its antimicrobial and anti-inflammatory properties effectively clean the blood and promote overall immune function.

Most Potent Method of Ingestion

The most effective way to use Red Root is as a tincture or tea. The tincture provides a concentrated dose of the active compounds, while the tea allows for gentle detoxification over time. It is often combined with other herbs that support lymphatic health for a more comprehensive detox regimen. As a tincture, take 1–2 ml three times daily. For tea, drink 1–2 cups a day to support lymphatic and detoxification processes.

Simple Recipe: Red Root Detox Tea

Add 1 teaspoon of dried Red Root to a cup. Pour boiling water over the herb and steep for 10 minutes. Strain and sip throughout the day to cleanse the lymphatic system and support detoxification.

Best Herbs to Use Together

Red Root works well with cleavers and burdock root. Cleavers enhances lymphatic drainage, while burdock root provides additional detoxifying and blood-purifying benefits.

116. Oregon Grape Root (*Mahonia aquifolium*)

Historical Context

Oregon grape root, named after the distinctive spiny leaves resembling holly, has been used for centuries by Native American tribes in the Pacific Northwest. This herb has a rich history of use for its antimicrobial and purifying qualities, particularly in supporting liver health and improving the body's ability to eliminate toxins. Early settlers adopted Oregon grape root as a natural remedy for skin conditions, digestive issues, and liver disorders.

Active Compounds and Benefits

Oregon grape root contains berberine, a potent alkaloid known for its antimicrobial, anti-inflammatory, and immune-supporting properties. Berberine helps to cleanse the liver, improve bile flow, and enhance the body's ability to process and eliminate toxins. The root also contains tannins, which have astringent qualities, helping to tighten tissues and support the detoxification of the gastrointestinal tract.

Most Potent Method of Ingestion

Oregon grape root is most effective when taken as a tincture or decoction. The tincture delivers the active compounds directly into the bloodstream, while the decoction allows for a gentle, prolonged cleansing effect. For a tincture, take 1–2 ml three times a day. For a decoction, drink 1–2 times a day to promote detoxification.

Simple Recipe: Oregon Grape Root Detox Decoction

Place 1–2 teaspoons of dried Oregon grape root in a pot with 1 cup of water. Simmer for 10–15 minutes, then strain. Drink once or twice a day to support liver detoxification and cleanse the body of toxins.

Best Herbs to Use Together

Combine Oregon grape root with dandelion root and milk thistle. Dandelion root enhances liver detoxification, while milk thistle protects liver cells from oxidative stress.

ANTI-INFLAMMATORY IMMUNITY BOOSTERS

117. Agrimony (*Agrimonia eupatoria*)

Historical Context

Agrimony has long been a staple herb in European herbal traditions. Often called "church steeples" due to its tall, spike-like flower clusters, agrimony has been used as a remedy for inflammatory conditions since the ancient Greeks. Agrimony was highly regarded for its ability to reduce swelling and inflammation, and it found its place in treatments for digestive issues, liver health, and respiratory ailments. Early herbalists also believed that agrimony had protective and purifying properties, both physically and spiritually.

Active Compounds and Benefits

Agrimony contains flavonoids, tannins, and phenolic acids that give it potent anti-inflammatory and immune-boosting qualities. Agrimony also supports the liver and kidneys, encouraging the removal of toxins from the body and improving overall immune function. Its mild astringent properties contribute to its ability to tighten tissues and tone the body, making it effective in treating inflammation-related conditions.

Most Potent Method of Ingestion

Agrimony is most effective as an infusion or tincture. The tincture provides a concentrated dose, while the infusion gently supports long-term immune function and inflammation reduction. Agrimony can also be used in combination with other anti-inflammatory herbs for enhanced effects. Take 1–2 ml three times daily as a tincture. For an infusion, drink 1–2 cups a day to help reduce inflammation and support immunity.

Simple Recipe: Agrimony Immune-Boosting Infusion

Place 1–2 teaspoons of dried agrimony in a cup. Pour boiling water over the herb and steep for 10–15 minutes. Strain and enjoy 1–2 cups daily to support inflammation reduction and immune function.

Best Herbs to Use Together

Agrimony pairs well with echinacea for an enhanced immune-boosting effect. Echinacea stimulates the immune system, while agrimony reduces inflammation, providing a balanced approach to strengthening immunity and addressing chronic inflammation.

118. Black Walnut (*Juglans nigra*)

Historical Context

Black walnut has long been a revered herb among Native American tribes, who utilized its powerful properties for cleansing and anti-inflammatory support. The tree, known for its deeply grooved bark and large, nutritious nuts, was traditionally used to treat everything from digestive issues to skin conditions. Black walnut's strong reputation as an anti-parasitic and immune-boosting herb has earned it a place in modern herbalism.

Active Compounds and Benefits

Black walnut contains juglone, a potent compound with powerful anti-inflammatory, antiparasitic, and antimicrobial properties. Juglone helps reduce inflammation, particularly in the digestive system. Black walnut's antimicrobial properties also support the immune system by fighting off infections and boosting the body's defenses against pathogens. Additionally, its tannins provide astringent benefits, which help tone the digestive tract and support overall health.

Most Potent Method of Ingestion

Black walnut is best used in tincture or capsule form, both of which provide a concentrated and effective dose of the active compounds. The tincture is especially useful for addressing inflammation quickly, while capsules offer a longer-lasting effect. For a tincture, take 1–2 ml three times daily. For capsules, follow the recommended dosage on the label, typically 300–500 mg per day. Adjust based on personal health needs.

Simple Recipe: Black Walnut Immune-Boosting Tincture

Place dried black walnut hulls in a glass jar and cover with high-proof alcohol. Seal the jar and store it in a cool, dark place for 4–6 weeks, shaking occasionally. Strain and take 1–2 ml three times a day to reduce inflammation and support immunity.

Best Herbs to Use Together

Combine black walnut with goldenseal for enhanced antimicrobial and anti-inflammatory effects. Goldenseal, with its powerful antibacterial properties, pairs perfectly with black walnut to support immune health and reduce inflammation in the body.

ADAPTOGENS FOR IMMUNE HEALTH

119. Ginkgo (*Ginkgo biloba*)

Historical Context

Ginkgo biloba, commonly known as "ginkgo" is one of the oldest living tree species and has a rich history of medicinal use in both Eastern and Western traditions. Known as a "living fossil," ginkgo has been used in traditional Chinese medicine for over a thousand years to improve circulation, support brain function, and promote vitality. Its leaves have been treasured for their ability to help the body adapt to stress, boost energy levels, and enhance immune function, making it a popular choice among those seeking to strengthen their resilience to illness.

Active Compounds and Benefits

Ginkgo is packed with powerful antioxidants, including flavonoids and terpenoids, which help combat oxidative stress and protect the immune system from damage. These compounds improve blood flow, which enhances oxygen and nutrient delivery throughout the body, including to immune cells, making the immune system more responsive. Additionally, ginkgo has adaptogenic properties, helping the body adapt to physical, mental, and environmental stress.

Most Potent Method of Ingestion

Ginkgo is most effective when taken as a standardized extract, typically in capsule or tincture form. This allows for the most consistent and potent delivery of its active compounds. A well-prepared extract ensures optimal absorption and long-lasting benefits for immune function. Take 120–240 mg of ginkgo extract per day, divided into 2–3 doses. This dosage range helps to improve circulation, support the immune system, and enhance overall energy levels.

Simple Recipe: Ginkgo Immune Support Tincture

Place 1 ounce of dried ginkgo leaves in a glass jar. Cover the leaves with high-proof alcohol (vodka or brandy). Seal and store in a cool, dark place for 4–6 weeks, shaking occasionally. Strain and take 1–2 ml of tincture up to three times daily to support immune health.

Best Herbs to Use Together

Ginkgo and astragalus combine well to bolster the body's defenses. While ginkgo improves circulation and boosts energy, astragalus enhances the immune system's overall resilience.

120. Spikenard (*Nardostachys jatamansi*)

Historical Context

Spikenard, also known as "nard," has been cherished for thousands of years, mentioned in both the Bible and ancient Ayurvedic texts. In traditional medicine, it was revered as a powerful adaptogen and tonic for the nervous system, promoting peace of mind, relaxation, and overall vitality. Spikenard was also used in rituals and as a perfume, which was believed to purify the spirit and promote a sense of grounding. In herbal practices, its immune-boosting and stress-reducing properties have been highly valued.

Active Compounds and Benefits

Spikenard contains the essential oils nardal and jatamansone, which possess potent anti-inflammatory, antioxidant, and immune-enhancing properties. These compounds help to regulate the body's response to stress and reduce inflammation, both of which are key to maintaining a strong immune system. As an adaptogen, spikenard improves the body's ability to cope with both physical and emotional stress, enhancing the immune system's efficiency in the face of illness.

Most Potent Method of Ingestion

The best way to consume spikenard for immune health is in the form of an extract or powder, because it allows for more concentrated and controlled doses. Spikenard's grounding properties are best supported when used in a daily regimen, either as a tea or in capsule form. For spikenard extract, take 1–2 ml of tincture daily, or if using the powdered root, take 500–1,000 mg per day. These dosages will support the body's natural resistance to stress and strengthen immune defenses over time.

Simple Recipe: Spikenard Immune-Boosting Tea

Add 1 teaspoon of dried spikenard root to 1 cup of boiling water. Steep for 10–15 minutes. Strain and sip on this soothing tea once or twice daily to boost immunity and manage stress.

Best Herbs to Use Together

Spikenard pairs wonderfully with ashwagandha, another adaptogen known for its ability to improve stress resilience and support overall vitality.

HERBS FOR
CARDIOVASCULAR HEALTH

LOWERING BLOOD PRESSURE

121. Hawthorn (*Crataegus monogyna*)

Historical Context

Hawthorn has a long history of being used as a cardiac tonic, with ancient Greek and Roman herbalists utilizing it to support heart health. Known as the "heart herb," hawthorn was first used in Europe as a remedy for heart disease, circulatory issues, and high blood pressure. In traditional medicine, this herb is cherished for its ability to strengthen the heart and improve circulation.

Active Compounds and Benefits

Hawthorn is rich in flavonoids, oligomeric proanthocyanidins (OPCs), and triterpenes, compounds known for their antioxidant and anti-inflammatory effects. These bioactive compounds help to dilate blood vessels, improve blood flow, and support the cardiovascular system. Hawthorn has been shown to reduce high blood pressure by acting as a vasodilator, enhancing circulation and easing the strain on the heart. It also strengthens the heart muscle, improving its efficiency in pumping blood.

Most Potent Method of Ingestion

Hawthorn is most potent when consumed as a tincture, extract, or capsule, which delivers its active compounds in concentrated form. The tincture or extract offers the most bioavailable form, ensuring faster absorption. Take 300–600 mg of hawthorn extract daily, or 1–2 ml of hawthorn tincture up to three times per day to help regulate blood pressure and support cardiovascular health.

Simple Recipe: Hawthorn Blood Pressure Support Tincture

Place 1 ounce of dried hawthorn berries in a glass jar. Cover with high-proof alcohol (vodka or brandy). Seal the jar and store in a cool, dark place for 4–6 weeks, shaking occasionally. Strain and take 1–2 ml of tincture up to three times daily to support heart health.

Best Herbs to Use Together

Hawthorn pairs well with motherwort, which also helps regulate blood pressure by calming the nervous system and enhancing circulation.

122. Mistletoe (*Viscum album*)

Historical Context

Mistletoe has long been revered for its healing properties, with its use dating back to ancient Celtic and Druidic traditions. The Druids believed that mistletoe had magical properties that could heal the heart and promote longevity. In traditional European medicine, it was commonly used to treat circulatory problems, high blood pressure, and even heart conditions.

Active Compounds and Benefits

Mistletoe contains viscotoxin and other bioactive compounds that have a vasodilatory effect, helping to relax blood vessels and lower blood pressure. The herb's alkaloids and flavonoids are known for improving circulation, reducing stress, and supporting the heart by toning the vascular system. Mistletoe also acts as a mild sedative, helping to calm the nervous system and lowering stress-induced high blood pressure.

Most Potent Method of Ingestion

Mistletoe is most effective when used as a tincture or extract, which ensures the maximum concentration of its active compounds. For effective blood pressure support, take 1–2 ml of mistletoe tincture up to three times daily or 250–500 mg of mistletoe extract in capsule form.

Simple Recipe: Mistletoe Blood Pressure Tincture

Place 1 ounce of dried mistletoe leaves in a glass jar. Cover with high-proof alcohol (vodka or brandy).

Seal and store in a cool, dark place for 4–6 weeks, shaking occasionally. Strain and take 1–2 ml of tincture up to three times daily to support heart health.

Best Herbs to Use Together

Mistletoe works synergistically with hawthorn to regulate blood pressure and improve heart function. While mistletoe calms the heart and blood vessels, hawthorn strengthens the heart muscle, offering a well-rounded approach to cardiovascular support.

IMPROVING CIRCULATION

123. Mugwort (*Artemisia vulgaris*)

Historical Context

Mugwort, also known as its Latin name *Artemisia* after the Greek goddess Artemis, has been employed since ancient times in Chinese, Greek, and Native American medicine. Historically, it was used to treat a variety of ailments, including poor circulation, digestive issues, and menstrual discomfort. Its role in stimulating the flow of blood and qi (vital energy) made it particularly valuable for those seeking to support cardiovascular health.

Active Compounds and Benefits

Mugwort contains flavonoids, essential oils (such as thujone), and tannins, which give it its circulatory benefits. These compounds work together to stimulate blood flow, especially to the extremities, and to improve the overall efficiency of the cardiovascular system. By promoting circulation and blood oxygenation, mugwort helps reduce symptoms of poor circulation, such as cold hands and feet, fatigue, and stiffness. It also has anti-inflammatory properties, which help reduce swelling and ease discomfort from poor circulation.

Most Potent Method of Ingestion

Mugwort is most effective when used as a tincture or in an herbal steam inhalation. The tincture provides quick absorption and can be taken regularly to support circulation, while the steam helps open the airways and invigorate the circulatory system. Take 1–2 ml of mugwort tincture up to three times daily. For a circulatory boost, use a steam inhalation by adding 1–2 drops of mugwort essential oil to hot water and inhaling the steam for 5–10 minutes.

Simple Recipe: Mugwort Circulation-Boosting Tea

Steep 1–2 teaspoons of dried mugwort leaves in 1 cup of hot water for 10–15 minutes. Strain and drink 1–2 times daily to support circulation.

Best Herbs to Use Together

Mugwort pairs well with ginger, because both herbs promote blood flow. While mugwort focuses on stimulating circulation to the extremities, ginger warms the body, enhances blood circulation, and promotes overall heart health.

124. Self-Heal (*Prunella vulgaris*)

Historical Context

Self-Heal, also known as "Heal-All," is a traditional herb used in Europe, Asia, and North America for its restorative and healing qualities. This herb was historically used to treat wounds, bruises, and other ailments. In Chinese medicine, it was employed for liver, skin, and circulation conditions. Its use for improving blood flow and promoting overall vitality made it a staple in herbal medicine for boosting circulation.

Active Compounds and Benefits

Self-Heal is rich in tannins, flavonoids, and rosmarinic acid, which have anti-inflammatory, antioxidant, and circulatory-stimulating effects. These compounds help strengthen capillaries, improve blood flow, and reduce swelling, especially in the extremities. Self-Heal is also known for its ability to promote tissue repair, making it a wonderful herb for those recovering from injuries, swelling, or poor circulation. Additionally, it can help balance the body's fluids and promote detoxification.

Most Potent Method of Ingestion

Self-Heal is most potent when taken as a tincture or decoction. The tincture delivers a concentrated dose of the herb's active compounds, while the decoction offers a nourishing and healing approach. Take 1–2 ml of Self-Heal tincture up to three times daily. For a more potent effect, use a decoction once or twice daily.

Simple Recipe: Self-Heal Circulation Decoction

Boil 1–2 teaspoons of dried Self-Heal in 2 cups of water for 15–20 minutes. Strain and drink 1 cup daily to improve circulation and promote healing.

Best Herbs to Use Together

Self-Heal works synergistically with garlic, which enhances circulation and supports heart health. Together, they help reduce inflammation, improve blood flow, and promote overall cardiovascular wellness.

REDUCING CHOLESTEROL

125. Sea Buckthorn (*Hippophae rhamnoides*)

Historical Context

Sea buckthorn is a hardy shrub with vibrant orange berries. It has been used in traditional medicine for centuries, particularly in Tibetan, Chinese, and Russian herbal practices. Known for its ability to nourish and restore vitality, sea buckthorn has long been associated with promoting heart health. Ancient healers used it to treat a variety of conditions, from digestive issues to skin ailments. In modern herbalism, this herb has gained attention for supporting cardiovascular health, especially in managing cholesterol levels.

Active Compounds and Benefits

Sea buckthorn is rich in essential fatty acids, particularly omega-7, which help regulate cholesterol levels and support heart health. Its antioxidant-rich profile, including flavonoids and vitamin C, further supports cardiovascular health by reducing oxidative stress and preventing the buildup of harmful LDL cholesterol in the arteries. Sea buckthorn's high content of plant sterols also aids in reducing cholesterol absorption in the gut, leading to lower overall cholesterol levels in the bloodstream. Its anti-inflammatory properties help reduce arterial inflammation, further promoting heart health.

Most Potent Method of Ingestion

Sea buckthorn is most potent when taken as an oil or extract. The oil, rich in omega fatty acids, is also ideal for promoting skin health, offering a dual benefit. Take 1–2 teaspoons of sea buckthorn oil daily or use 1–2 ml of sea buckthorn extract. Consistent use is recommended for optimal cholesterol support.

Simple Recipe: Sea Buckthorn Heart Health Oil

Gently massage sea buckthorn oil onto the chest area or the soles of the feet to support circulation and heart health. Alternatively, add 1 teaspoon of sea buckthorn oil to smoothies or salads.

Best Herbs to Use Together

Sea buckthorn pairs well with hawthorn, a well-known heart tonic, to enhance cardiovascular benefits. Together, they support reducing cholesterol, improving circulation, and nourishing the heart.

126. Fo-Ti (*Polygonum multiflorum*)

Historical Context

Fo-Ti, also known as "He Shou Wu," has been a staple in traditional Chinese medicine (TCM) for over a thousand years. Historically, it was used to promote longevity, restore vitality, and rejuvenate the body. This herb has been particularly associated with kidney, liver, and cardiovascular health. In TCM, it is considered a "tonic herb," and it is believed to support the body in maintaining a healthy balance of energy. Its reputation for longevity and vitality has made it a prized herb for those seeking to reduce the signs of aging and improve overall health.

Active Compounds and Benefits

Fo-Ti contains compounds like stilbenes and resveratrol, which are known for their antioxidant properties. These compounds help reduce oxidative stress, lower cholesterol levels, and support overall heart health. Fo-Ti also contains alkaloids and flavonoids that help regulate lipid metabolism, making it a potent herb for reducing high cholesterol levels. Additionally, Fo-Ti supports liver and kidney health, which are vital for the body's natural detoxification processes and cholesterol regulation.

Most Potent Method of Ingestion

Fo-Ti is best used as an extract or in a powdered form. The extract is highly concentrated and effective for maintaining healthy cholesterol levels, while the powder can be added to smoothies or capsules for a more holistic approach. Take 1–2 grams of Fo-Ti powder daily or 1–2 ml of Fo-Ti extract. Since it is a tonic herb, it is most effective when used regularly over time.

Simple Recipe: Fo-Ti Cholesterol Support Smoothie

Blend 1 teaspoon of Fo-Ti powder with 1 cup of almond milk, 1 banana, and a handful of spinach.

Drink once a day to support healthy cholesterol levels.

Best Herbs to Use Together

Fo-Ti works well with turmeric, an anti-inflammatory herb that supports liver function and cholesterol metabolism. Together, they create a potent combination for managing cholesterol and improving cardiovascular health.

SUPPORTING HEART FUNCTION

127. Saffron (*Crocus sativus*)

Historical Context

Saffron, often referred to as "the golden spice," has a long history of use in both culinary and medicinal traditions. Traced back to ancient Persia, India, and Greece, saffron was valued not only for its unique flavor but also for its healing properties. In ancient times, it was used to treat a range of ailments, from digestive issues to mood disorders. Saffron's reputation in modern herbalism has grown, especially for its ability to support heart health by improving circulation.

Active Compounds and Benefits

The key active compounds in saffron, including crocin, safranal, and picrocrocin, are powerful antioxidants that support heart health by reducing oxidative stress and preventing plaque buildup in the arteries. These compounds have anti-inflammatory properties, which can reduce the risk of heart disease and stroke by promoting healthy blood circulation and preventing arterial damage. Saffron also helps regulate blood pressure, making it an ideal herb for maintaining overall heart function.

Most Potent Method of Ingestion

Saffron is most effective when used in extract form or as a tea. The extract, rich in bioactive compounds, provides targeted cardiovascular benefits, while a daily infusion can support long-term heart health. For consistent heart support, take 30–50 mg of saffron extract daily or drink saffron tea once a day.

Simple Recipe: Saffron Heart Health Tea

Steep 10–20 threads of saffron in a cup of hot water for 10 minutes. Drink once daily to support circulation and heart function.

Best Herbs to Use Together

Saffron works well with hawthorn, a well-known herb for strengthening heart function.

128. Red Date (*Ziziphus jujuba*)

Historical Context

Ziziphus, or red date, also known as "Jujube," has been used for over 4,000 years in traditional Chinese medicine (TCM) to treat various health issues. Revered as a tonic herb, red date was often used to restore vitality, improve sleep, and support cardiovascular health. It has long been considered a symbol of longevity and strength, often recommended for elderly individuals to enhance heart function and overall well-being.

Active Compounds and Benefits

Red date contains saponins, flavonoids, and alkaloids, all of which contribute to its heart-boosting benefits. These compounds are known for regulating blood pressure, improving circulation, and strengthening heart function. Red date helps lower cholesterol levels, reducing the risk of atherosclerosis, while its sedative properties help reduce stress and anxiety, which are often contributors to heart disease. Additionally, its ability to improve sleep supports overall heart health.

Most Potent Method of Ingestion

Red date is most effective in extract form, which provides concentrated support for heart health and stress reduction. It can also be consumed as a decoction for those seeking a soothing, restorative remedy. Take 1–2 ml of red date extract daily or brew 1-2 teaspoons of dried red date fruit in water to make a decoction. Drink 1–2 times a day to support cardiovascular function and reduce stress.

Simple Recipe: Ziziphus Heart Tonic Decoction

Add 1–2 teaspoons of dried red date fruit to 1 cup of water. Bring to a boil, then simmer for 10–15 minutes. Drink daily to calm the mind and promote heart health.

Best Herbs to Use Together

Red date pairs well with Schisandra, another adaptogenic herb, to support heart health, reduce stress, and enhance vitality. Together, they offer a potent combination for promoting long-term cardiovascular wellness and overall resilience.

MANAGING HEART PALPITATIONS

129. Wood Betony (*Stachys officinalis*)

Historical Context

Wood betony, also known as "betony" or "purple betony," has a rich history in European herbalism, where it was considered a cure-all by medieval herbalists. It was used to treat a range of ailments, from headaches to digestive disorders. Among its many uses, wood betony was particularly valued for its ability to ease anxiety, soothe the nervous system, and support heart health, especially in managing heart palpitations caused by stress or emotional turmoil.

Active Compounds and Benefits

Wood betony is rich in flavonoids, tannins, and essential oils, which provide its sedative, anti-inflammatory, and heart-strengthening effects. Its nervine qualities make it ideal for calming the nervous system, which is crucial for preventing the anxiety-induced palpitations that often accompany stress. The herb also supports blood flow and helps regulate the heart's rhythm. By balancing the autonomic nervous system, wood betony aids in preventing arrhythmias and fluttering sensations that can cause discomfort.

Most Potent Method of Ingestion

The most effective form of wood betony is a tincture. A warm infusion can also benefit those seeking a relaxing, soothing remedy before bed or during moments of stress. Take 1–2 ml of wood betony tincture up to three times a day or steep 1–2 teaspoons of dried herb in hot water to make an infusion. Drink 1–2 times daily for long-term heart support.

Simple Recipe: Wood Betony Heart Relaxing Tincture

Fill a jar with fresh or dried wood betony leaves and flowers. Cover with high-proof alcohol (vodka or brandy). Seal and store in a cool, dark place for 4–6 weeks, shaking occasionally. Strain and take 1–2 ml up to three times a day to support heart rhythm and calm nervous tension.

Best Herbs to Use Together

Wood betony pairs well with hawthorn, a classic heart tonic, for additional support in regulating heart palpitations and promoting overall heart health.

130. Chinese Date (*Ziziphus spinosa*)

Historical Context

Chinese date, also known as "Jujube," has been utilized for centuries in traditional Chinese medicine (TCM) to treat various conditions, particularly those related to the heart and nervous system. Known for its calming, sedative properties, it has long been used to treat insomnia, anxiety, and palpitations, all of which are often linked to an overactive heart and stressful lifestyle.

Active Compounds and Benefits

Chinese date contains alkaloids, flavonoids, and saponins that work together to calm the nervous system, reduce stress, and support heart function. These compounds help to stabilize the heartbeat and reduce the occurrence of palpitations, particularly those triggered by emotional stress or anxiety. Chinese date is also known to nourish the blood and improve circulation, enhancing overall cardiovascular function. Its mild sedative effects help alleviate the anxiety that often accompanies heart palpitations.

Most Potent Method of Ingestion

Chinese date is most potent when taken in the form of an extract or decoction. The extract allows for concentrated support of heart health and nervous system calm, while the decoction offers a gentle, restorative approach. Take 1–2 ml of Chinese date extract daily or prepare a decoction and drink it 1–2 times a day to help reduce heart palpitations and promote relaxation.

Simple Recipe: Ziziphus Calming Decoction

Add 1–2 teaspoons of dried Chinese date fruit to 1 cup of water. Bring to a boil, then simmer for 10–15 minutes. Drink once or twice a day to reduce palpitations and calm the heart.

Best Herbs to Use Together

Chinese date works synergistically with wood betony to enhance the calming effects on the nervous system and heart.

REDUCING INFLAMMATION IN BLOOD VESSELS

131. Tansy (*Tanacetum vulgare*)

Historical Context

Tansy, also known as "mother of thousands," has a long-standing tradition in European herbalism, where it was used for a variety of ailments, including digestive issues, parasites, and menstrual discomfort. Although lesser known today, it was once highly regarded for its ability to stimulate circulation and reduce inflammation. In particular, tansy was used to treat conditions involving inflammation in the blood vessels.

Active Compounds and Benefits

Tansy contains potent compounds such as flavonoids, sesquiterpene lactones, and tannins that help to reduce inflammation and support vascular health. These compounds work together to soothe inflammation within the blood vessels, reduce swelling, and improve blood flow. Tansy also has a mild analgesic effect, which can help reduce the pain that often accompanies vascular inflammation. It is also an excellent herb for managing conditions like varicose veins and arterial inflammation.

Most Potent Method of Ingestion

Tansy is most effective when taken as a tincture or in a topical infusion. A tincture offers quick absorption and concentrated relief, while an infusion can be soothing and beneficial for long-term vascular health. Take 1–2 ml of tansy tincture up to three times a day or steep 1–2 teaspoons of dried tansy leaves in hot water to make an infusion. Drink 1–2 times daily for ongoing support.

Simple Recipe: Tansy Vascular Health Tincture

Place dried tansy flowers and leaves in a glass jar. Cover with high-proof alcohol (vodka or brandy). Seal and store in a cool, dark place for 4–6 weeks, shaking occasionally. Strain and take 1–2 ml up to three times a day to support blood vessel health and reduce inflammation.

Best Herbs to Use Together

Tansy works well with horse chestnut, a known remedy for improving circulation and reducing inflammation in the veins, providing a synergistic approach to vascular health.

132. Fringe Tree (*Chionanthus virginicus*)

Historical Context

Fringe tree, also called "white fringe tree" or "Old Man's Beard," is native to the Southeastern United States and has been used in traditional herbal practices by Native American tribes for its detoxifying and anti-inflammatory properties. Often employed to treat liver conditions and support the lymphatic system, fringe tree has more recently gained attention for its ability to support cardiovascular health by reducing inflammation in the blood vessels.

Active Compounds and Benefits

Fringe tree contains iridoid glycosides, flavonoids, and lignans, compounds that have demonstrated potent anti-inflammatory effects. These compounds specifically help to target inflammation within the vascular system, improving blood flow and reducing the risk of vascular damage. Fringe tree also has mild diuretic properties, which can assist with fluid retention that may contribute to vascular inflammation. This herb is particularly beneficial for individuals dealing with conditions such as arteriosclerosis, poor circulation, and inflammation in the veins.

Most Potent Method of Ingestion

The most effective way to consume fringe tree is through an extract or tincture, which allows the active compounds to be absorbed quickly and provide long-lasting benefits for vascular health. Take 1–2 ml of fringe tree extract or tincture up to three times a day. For long-term support, it can also be taken as part of a daily regimen.

Simple Recipe: Fringe Tree Vascular Health Tincture

Fill a jar with dried fringe tree bark and leaves. Cover with high-proof alcohol (vodka or brandy).

Seal and store in a cool, dark place for 4–6 weeks, shaking occasionally. Strain and take 1–2 ml up to three times a day to reduce vascular inflammation and improve circulation.

Best Herbs to Use Together

Fringe tree pairs well with ginkgo, an herb known for its circulation-boosting properties. Together, they can offer powerful support for overall cardiovascular health.

SUPPORTING HEALTHY BLOOD VESSELS

133. Dill (*Anethum graveolens*)

Historical Context

Dill is an aromatic herb with a long history in both culinary and medicinal traditions. It has been valued since ancient times for its ability to aid digestion, relieve colic, and support overall health. In ancient Greece, dill was often used to soothe digestive issues and promote relaxation. Traditional herbalists recognized its beneficial effects on blood vessels and utilized its soothing properties to ease circulatory problems.

Active Compounds and Benefits

Dill contains the essential oils carvone and limonene, plus flavonoids and coumarins, which contribute to its anti-inflammatory and antioxidant effects. These compounds help protect the blood vessels from oxidative damage and reduce inflammation within the vascular walls. Dill also acts as a mild diuretic, supporting the elimination of excess fluid from the body and reducing the strain on blood vessels. Its ability to promote circulation and soothe vascular inflammation makes it an ideal herb for supporting blood vessel health.

Most Potent Method of Ingestion

Dill is best consumed as an infusion or tincture, which allows for the absorption of its active compounds. The infusion provides a gentle and soothing remedy, while the tincture delivers a more concentrated dose for long-lasting effects. Drink dill infusion up to two times a day. Alternatively, take 1–2 ml of dill tincture up to three times daily for a more concentrated effect.

Simple Recipe: Dill Vascular Support Infusion

Place 1–2 teaspoons of dried dill seeds in a teapot or infuser. Pour boiling water over the seeds and steep for 5–10 minutes. Strain and enjoy the infusion to help soothe and support healthy blood vessels.

Best Herbs to Use Together

Dill pairs well with hawthorn, a well-known herb for supporting heart health and improving circulation. Together, they can help strengthen the blood vessels and promote overall cardiovascular well-being.

134. Cardamom (*Elettaria cardamomum*)

Historical Context

Cardamom, often referred to as the "Queen of Spices," has been a treasured herb in Ayurvedic medicine for thousands of years. It is known for its warming and aromatic properties and has been used to treat a variety of digestive issues, respiratory ailments, and circulatory problems. In traditional medicine, cardamom was often prescribed to improve circulation, relieve bloating, and support healthy blood flow, making it a valuable herb for promoting vascular health.

Active Compounds and Benefits

Cardamom contains the essential oils cineole, terpinene, and α-terpinyl acetate, which contribute to its anti-inflammatory and antioxidant properties. These compounds help reduce oxidative stress within the blood vessels and promote blood circulation. Cardamom is also known for its ability to improve endothelial function, which is essential for maintaining blood vessels' flexibility and health. Its gentle diuretic effect further supports healthy blood pressure by reducing excess fluid in the body.

Most Potent Method of Ingestion

The most effective way to consume cardamom is in powder or extract form. The powder can be added to beverages or used in cooking, while the extract provides a concentrated dose that supports cardiovascular health.

Simple Recipe: Cardamom Vascular Health Tea

Add 1 teaspoon of ground cardamom to a cup of tea. Let it steep for 5 minutes, then strain and enjoy. Drink once or twice a day to support healthy blood vessels and improve circulation. Alternatively, take 1–2 ml of cardamom extract up to twice daily.

Best Herbs to Use Together

Cardamom combines well with cinnamon, another circulatory tonic, to provide a powerful combination that enhances blood flow, reduces inflammation, and supports the overall health of the blood vessels.

MANAGING VARICOSE VEINS

135. Onion (*Allium cepa*)

Historical Context

Onion, a humble kitchen staple, has long been celebrated for its medicinal properties across cultures. In ancient Egypt, it was used not only as a food but also as a remedy for a variety of ailments. The powerful medicinal properties of onions were further recognized in Europe, where folk medicine used them to treat circulatory problems and inflammation. In modern herbalism, onion extract is increasingly valued for managing varicose veins.

Active Compounds and Benefits

Onion extract is rich in sulfur compounds like quercetin and diallyl disulfide, which are known for their anti-inflammatory, antioxidant, and circulatory-stimulating properties. These compounds help reduce inflammation in the veins, improve blood circulation, and strengthen the walls of blood vessels.

Most Potent Method of Ingestion

Onion extract is most effective in tincture or capsule form, allowing for concentrated absorption of its beneficial compounds. Take 1–2 ml of onion extract tincture up to three times daily, or follow the dosage instructions provided on the supplement label. Onion extract capsules are also available, with a typical dose of 300–500 mg, taken twice a day.

Simple Recipe: Onion Extract Vein Support Tincture

Peel and chop a medium-sized onion and place it in a glass jar. Cover with high-proof alcohol, such as vodka, ensuring the onion is fully submerged. Seal the jar and store it in a cool, dark place for 4–6 weeks, shaking it every few days. Strain and take 1–2 ml of the tincture up to three times a day to promote healthy circulation and manage varicose veins.

Best Herbs to Use Together

Combine onion extract with horse chestnut, an herb known for its ability to strengthen blood vessels and reduce swelling in varicose veins. Together, they form a synergistic formula for improving venous circulation and easing the discomfort of varicose veins.

136. Chickweed (*Stellaria media*)

Historical Context

Chickweed has long been a cherished herb in folk medicine, particularly in European and Native American traditions. This herb has been used for centuries to treat a variety of skin conditions, inflammation, and digestive complaints. Its benefits extend to vascular health, where it is used to alleviate the discomfort associated with varicose veins, swollen legs, and poor circulation.

Active Compounds and Benefits

Chickweed contains saponins, flavonoids, and vitamin C, which contribute to its anti-inflammatory, astringent, and circulatory-stimulating effects. These compounds help to reduce swelling, strengthen vein walls, and improve blood flow, making chickweed a valuable herb for managing varicose veins.

Most Potent Method of Ingestion

Chickweed is most effective when applied topically as a poultice or salve for localized relief, but it can also be consumed as an infusion or tincture to support systemic circulation and vascular health. For an infusion, steep 1–2 teaspoons of dried chickweed in hot water for 10–15 minutes. Drink 1–2 cups per day to support vein health. Alternatively, use chickweed tincture at a dose of 1–2 ml up to three times daily for stronger circulation support.

Simple Recipe: Chickweed Poultice for Varicose Veins

Place a handful of fresh chickweed leaves in a mortar and pestle or food processor, adding a little water to form a paste. Apply the paste directly to the varicose veins and cover with a clean cloth. Leave on for 20–30 minutes, then rinse off. Repeat daily to help reduce swelling and inflammation in the veins.

Best Herbs to Use Together

Chickweed pairs well with Gotu Kola, which is known for improving circulation and strengthening blood vessel walls. Together, they make an effective topical and internal remedy for varicose veins and venous insufficiency.

PREVENTING BLOOD CLOTS

137. Cranberry (*Vaccinium macrocarpon*)

Historical Context

Cranberry has a long-standing reputation as a health-boosting berry in both culinary and medicinal traditions. Native to North America, Indigenous tribes utilized cranberries for their potent antimicrobial and anti-inflammatory properties, often using them to treat urinary tract infections and support overall health. Modern herbalism has expanded its uses, with cranberry being recognized for preventing blood clots and supporting cardiovascular health.

Active Compounds and Benefits

Cranberry is rich in proanthocyanidins, antioxidants that play a crucial role in preventing the aggregation of platelets, which is essential for blood clot prevention. These compounds help inhibit the formation of clots while promoting healthy circulation. Cranberry also contains vitamin C.

Most Potent Method of Ingestion

Cranberry is most effective when consumed as a fresh juice, extract, or supplement. The concentrated form of cranberry in tinctures or capsules delivers a potent dose of its beneficial compounds. For prevention, regular consumption is key. Take 1–2 tablespoons of pure cranberry juice daily or 500–1,000 mg of cranberry extract two times per day. For those using cranberry capsules, the recommended dose is typically 400–800 mg per day, divided into two doses.

Simple Recipe: Cranberry Blood Flow Tincture

Place fresh or dried cranberries in a jar and cover with high-proof alcohol (such as vodka). Seal the jar and store it in a cool, dark place for 4–6 weeks, shaking occasionally. Strain the mixture and take 1–2 ml up to three times daily to promote healthy circulation and prevent blood clots.

Best Herbs to Use Together

Cranberry works synergistically with turmeric, which has strong anti-inflammatory properties and enhances circulation.

138. Avocado Oil (*from Persea americana*)

Historical Context

Avocado oil, derived from the pulp of the avocado fruit (*Persea Americana*), has been a staple in the diets and healing practices of Indigenous peoples in Central and South America for a long time. The oil was used both for its nutritional value and its medicinal properties and was revered for its ability to nourish the skin and support cardiovascular health. In recent years, its use has expanded in modern herbalism for preventing blood clots and promoting healthy circulation.

Active Compounds and Benefits

Avocado oil is rich in monounsaturated fats, particularly oleic acid, which has anti-inflammatory and anticoagulant properties. These healthy fats help to thin the blood, improving circulation and reducing the risk of clot formation. Additionally, avocado oil contains vitamin E, which supports blood vessel health by preventing oxidative stress and promoting elasticity in the walls of veins and arteries. This combination of fats and nutrients makes avocado oil an effective natural remedy for preventing blood clots.

Most Potent Method of Ingestion:

Avocado oil is most beneficial when consumed in its raw form as part of a daily diet, either as a cooking oil or as a dressing for salads. It can also be used as a supplement or in its pure form for topical applications to nourish the skin and support vascular health. Incorporate 1–2 tablespoons of avocado oil into your daily diet by using it in smoothies, salads, or as a cooking oil. For those using it for medicinal purposes, 500–1,000 mg of avocado oil supplement may be taken daily.

Simple Recipe: Avocado Oil-Infused Circulatory Balm

Mix 2 tablespoons of avocado oil with 1 tablespoon of cayenne pepper and a few drops of lavender essential oil. Gently warm the mixture and apply it topically to the legs or areas of concern for better circulation and to prevent blood clots. Massage the balm into the skin in circular motions, promoting smooth blood flow.

Best Herbs to Use Together

Avocado oil can be combined with ginger, which also promotes circulation and blood thinning. This creates a powerful remedy for preventing blood clots and improving overall cardiovascular health.

PROMOTING HEALTHY BLOOD SUGAR LEVELS

139. Cinnamon (*Cinnamomum verum*)

Historical Context

Cinnamon, often referred to as "the king of spices," has been prized for thousands of years in both culinary and medicinal traditions. Ancient Egyptians used it in embalming, while the Greeks and Romans believed it had powerful healing properties. Throughout history, cinnamon has been cherished not only for its sweet, warming flavor but also for its ability to regulate blood sugar and support metabolic health. Modern herbal medicine has well-documented cinnamon benefits for managing blood sugar levels.

Active Compounds and Benefits

Cinnamon contains bioactive compounds such as cinnamaldehyde, polyphenols, and flavonoids, which are known for their ability to regulate blood sugar levels. These compounds help improve insulin sensitivity by mimicking insulin's effects in the body, allowing cells to absorb glucose better. Additionally, cinnamon helps slow down carbohydrate digestion, preventing rapid spikes in blood sugar. Its antioxidant and anti-inflammatory properties further support overall metabolic health.

Most Potent Method of Ingestion

Cinnamon is most effective when consumed in powdered form, whether in teas, smoothies, or sprinkled over foods. Cinnamon extract or a tincture is also highly potent. For long-term use, it is best taken in combination with other blood-sugar-regulating herbs. For optimal blood sugar support, take 1–2 teaspoons of cinnamon powder per day, or 1–2 ml of cinnamon tincture 2–3 times daily. Be cautious not to exceed the recommended dose, because large amounts may cause digestive discomfort.

Simple Recipe: Cinnamon Blood Sugar Support Tea

Boil 1 cup of water and add 1 cinnamon stick or 1 teaspoon of ground cinnamon. Let it steep for 5–10 minutes. Drink the tea twice daily to help stabilize blood sugar levels.

Best Herbs to Use Together

Cinnamon pairs well with fenugreek, another herb known for its ability to regulate blood sugar levels. Together, they create a powerful duo for managing blood sugar and improving insulin sensitivity.

140. Cucumber (*Cucumis sativus*)

Historical Context

Native to India and prized in ancient civilizations such as Egypt and Greece, cucumber has been used for both its refreshing taste and its health benefits. In traditional medicine, cucumber was applied to soothe the skin, detoxify the body, and balance blood sugar levels. Today, it remains a popular remedy for promoting hydration and supporting overall metabolic health.

Active Compounds and Benefits

Cucumber is rich in antioxidants, particularly flavonoids and tannins, which help reduce oxidative stress and inflammation—two factors that can impact blood sugar regulation. Cucumber also contains a high percentage of water, which aids in hydration and supports kidney function, indirectly assisting in blood sugar management. Furthermore, the fruit has been shown to enhance insulin sensitivity, making it a helpful addition for those looking to balance their blood sugar levels naturally.

Most Potent Method of Ingestion

Cucumber is best consumed fresh, either as part of a salad, smoothie, or simply sliced as a snack. It can also be juiced for a refreshing, hydrating beverage that supports blood sugar balance. For maximum benefit, it's recommended to use organic cucumber to avoid pesticide residues. Consume 1 cup of sliced cucumber per day, either as part of a meal or as a snack. If juicing, half to a whole cucumber per day is ideal. You can also incorporate cucumber in your daily salads or smoothies.

Simple Recipe: Cucumber Blood Sugar–Regulator Smoothie

Blend 1 cup of cucumber slices, 1 small apple, half a teaspoon of cinnamon, and 1 tablespoon of lemon juice. Add water or coconut water to thin the smoothie, if desired. Drink daily to support healthy blood sugar levels.

Best Herbs to Use Together

Pair cucumber with bitter melon, which has similar blood-sugar-lowering effects. Together, they create a cooling, detoxifying remedy that helps maintain balanced blood sugar levels naturally.

HERBS FOR DETOXIFICATION

LIVER DETOXIFICATION

141. Chanca Piedra (*Phyllanthus niruri*)

Historical Context

Known as "stone breaker" in traditional herbalism, Chanca Piedra has a long history of use in South American medicine for its remarkable ability to support kidney and liver health. Indigenous peoples of the Amazon rainforest utilized this herb to treat liver disorders, cleanse the urinary system, and promote overall detoxification. In modern herbal practices, it has earned a reputation as a powerful liver detoxifier and is particularly renowned for its ability to break down kidney stones.

Active Compounds and Benefits

Chanca Piedra is rich in lignans, flavonoids, and alkaloids, which have powerful hepatoprotective (liver-protecting) properties. The herb promotes the elimination of toxins, reduces inflammation, and supports liver function by enhancing bile production and flow. Its active compounds also protect the liver from oxidative stress, making it a vital ally in liver detoxification. Additionally, Chanca Piedra is effective in reducing uric acid levels, which is beneficial for those struggling with liver-related ailments such as fatty liver disease or hepatitis.

Most Potent Method of Ingestion

Chanca Piedra is most effective as an herbal infusion or decoction. While tinctures can be helpful, the tea or decoction allows the liver to fully benefit from its detoxifying compounds. For a deeper, more concentrated effect, consider using the herb in extract form. For liver detoxification, drink Chanca Piedra tea up to three times daily. If using a tincture, take 1–2 ml three times a day. For long-term liver health support, use periodically, because prolonged use may overstimulate detoxification processes.

Simple Recipe: Chanca Piedra Liver Detox Tea

Boil 1 cup of water and add 1 teaspoon of dried Chanca Piedra. Steep for 10–15 minutes, then strain. Drink 1–2 cups daily to promote liver detoxification.

Best Herbs to Use Together

Combine Chanca Piedra with milk thistle for enhanced liver protection and detoxification. Milk thistle's silymarin works synergistically with Chanca Piedra to support liver cell regeneration and protect against toxins.

142. Bupleurum (*Bupleurum chinense*)

Historical Context

Bupleurum has been used for over two thousand years in traditional Chinese medicine (TCM) for its ability to regulate the liver and promote detoxification. Known as *chai hu* in Chinese medicine, bupleurum is a key herb in many classical TCM formulations aimed at enhancing liver function, improving circulation, and alleviating stress. Its use spans across treating liver disorders, detoxification, and even as a remedy for emotional imbalances related to the liver's role in regulating the body's qi (energy).

Active Compounds and Benefits

Bupleurum contains saponins, flavonoids, and lignans, which have significant hepatoprotective effects. The herb helps stimulate liver detoxification by promoting bile flow and liver qi movement, which is essential for detoxification and the body's overall metabolic function. Bupleurum also supports the immune system by reducing inflammation and promoting lymphatic drainage.

Most Potent Method of Ingestion

Bupleurum can best be taken as a decoction, which extracts its beneficial compounds more thoroughly. A tincture or extract can also be effective for a more concentrated dose, although the decoction offers a more holistic approach to liver detox. Take bupleurum root decoction or tea up to two times daily. For tinctures, 1–2 ml can be taken 2–3 times a day. It is advisable to cycle the herb for long-term use to prevent overstimulation.

Simple Recipe: Bupleurum Liver Detox Decoction

Boil 1 cup of water and add 1 teaspoon of dried bupleurum root. Let it simmer for 20–30 minutes.

Strain and drink 1 cup daily to support liver detoxification.

Best Herbs to Use Together

Combine bupleurum with Schisandra berry, another herb revered in TCM for its liver-strengthening and detoxifying properties. This combination enhances liver function and promotes the harmonious flow of qi, supporting both detoxification and energy levels.

KIDNEY SUPPORT

143. Cleavers (*Galium aparine*)

Historical Context

Cleavers, also known as "bedstraw," has been used since ancient times to support the lymphatic system and promote detoxification. It was popularized in medieval herbalism and in European folk medicine as a remedy for clearing waste from the kidneys and lymphatic tissues. Cleavers is often associated with cleansing and purifying herbs, traditionally used during fasting and spring detox regimens to support overall bodily function.

Active Compounds and Benefits

Cleavers contains flavonoids, glycosides, and tannins, which work together to stimulate the kidneys and lymphatic system. It has diuretic properties, increasing urine production to flush toxins from the body. Cleavers also supports the integrity of kidney tissues, helping to reduce inflammation and protect against kidney stone formation. The herb is gentle enough for long-term use to aid in mild kidney conditions and as a lymphatic cleanser.

Most Potent Method of Ingestion

Cleavers is most effectively consumed as a tincture or infusion. Its mild nature makes it suitable for use as a gentle diuretic in both forms. For individuals looking for a more concentrated remedy, a tincture offers a more direct and potent dose of its active compounds. For an infusion drink up to 2 cups daily. If using tincture form, take 1–2 ml three times a day. Cleavers can be safely used long-term for general kidney support.

Simple Recipe: Cleavers Kidney Detox Infusion

Steep 1–2 teaspoons of dried cleavers in 1 cup of boiling water for 10–15 minutes. Strain and enjoy up to two cups a day for kidney support.

Best Herbs to Use Together

Cleavers pairs well with dandelion root and nettle leaf for a kidney-cleansing formula. Dandelion root helps to cleanse the liver and kidneys, while nettle leaf supports urinary tract health, creating a balanced approach to kidney detoxification.

144. Corn Silk (*from Zea mays*)

Historical Context

Corn silk, the long, golden threads that grow from the top of an ear of corn (*Zea mays*), has been a prized herbal remedy in Native American and traditional European herbal medicine. It was historically used for its soothing properties on the urinary system and kidneys. Known for its mild diuretic effects, corn silk has been utilized for a variety of urinary issues, including kidney stones, infections, and inflammation.

Active Compounds and Benefits

Corn silk is rich in flavonoids, saponins, and alkaloids, all of which contribute to its diuretic, anti-inflammatory, and anti-spasmodic properties. The herb supports the kidneys by encouraging urine flow, which helps flush out toxins, reduce water retention, and ease inflammation. Corn silk is particularly beneficial in addressing conditions such as cystitis and mild kidney infections due to its soothing effect on the urinary tract lining.

Most Potent Method of Ingestion

Corn silk can be taken as an infusion, tincture, or even in capsule form for convenience. Its mild and gentle nature makes it especially suitable for infusions or teas, although a tincture can be beneficial for more potent action. Drink corn silk infusion up to 3 cups daily. For tincture use, take 1–2 ml up to three times per day. It is safe for long-term use, particularly for individuals with recurring urinary issues.

Simple Recipe: Corn Silk Kidney Tea

Steep 1–2 teaspoons of dried corn silk in 1 cup of boiling water for 10–15 minutes. Strain and enjoy 1–3 cups daily to support kidney function and urinary health.

Best Herbs to Use Together

Combine corn silk with marshmallow root and horsetail for a comprehensive kidney-supportive blend. Marshmallow root helps soothe irritation in the urinary tract, while horsetail provides additional minerals beneficial for kidney health, promoting overall urinary system wellness.

DIGESTIVE CLEANSING

145. Triphala *(combination of Emblica officinalis, Terminalia chebula, and Terminalia bellirica)*

Historical Context

Triphala, a revered formula in Ayurvedic medicine, is composed of three fruits: Amalaki (*Emblica officinalis*), Haritaki (*Terminalia chebula*), and Bibhitaki (*Terminalia bellirica*). This triad has been used for thousands of years to support digestion, detoxification, and overall vitality. In traditional practice, Triphala is often taken daily as part of a rejuvenating routine, promoting longevity and holistic balance by cleansing the digestive system and aiding nutrient absorption.

Active Compounds and Benefits

Each fruit in Triphala brings its own set of active compounds, working synergistically to enhance digestive health. Amalaki, rich in vitamin C and antioxidants, supports the digestive tract's ability to absorb nutrients while providing gentle laxative effects. Haritaki acts as a detoxifier, promoting bowel regularity and cleansing the colon. Bibhitaki helps to clear excess mucus and toxins from the body, particularly in the lungs and intestines. Together, they support optimal digestion, detoxification, and regularity.

Most Potent Method of Ingestion

Triphala is most commonly consumed as a powder or in tablet form. The powder can be mixed with warm water or taken with honey for easier consumption. For tablets, follow the manufacturer's recommended dose.

Simple Recipe: Triphala Digestive Cleansing Mix

Take 1 teaspoon of Triphala powder and mix it into a glass of warm water before bedtime. Drink regularly to cleanse and rejuvenate the digestive system.

Best Herbs to Use Together

Combine Triphala with ginger and fennel to enhance digestive cleansing. Ginger aids digestion by stimulating gastric juices, while fennel supports detoxification and reduces bloating, creating a well-rounded digestive support formula.

146. Psyllium (*Plantago ovata*)

Historical Context

Psyllium has been used in traditional medicine for centuries, especially in the Middle East and India. Its ability to soothe the digestive system and provide gentle, natural fiber has earned it a place as a key remedy for constipation and digestive cleansing. Psyllium husk is most often used to promote bowel regularity and help detoxify the colon, offering support for healthy elimination and gut health.

Active Compounds and Benefits

Psyllium is rich in soluble fiber, which absorbs water and forms a gel-like substance in the intestines. This helps bulk up stool and promote regular bowel movements. It also supports overall gut health by acting as a prebiotic, feeding beneficial gut bacteria. Psyllium's ability to regulate the digestive process makes it an excellent aid for constipation, as well as for managing mild diarrhea by absorbing excess water.

Most Potent Method of Ingestion

Psyllium is most commonly consumed in powder or husk form. It can be added to water, smoothies, or soups, or taken in capsules for a more concentrated dosage. When taken, it is important to drink plenty of water to avoid dehydration or constipation. The dosage may vary depending on individual needs, but it is crucial to drink enough fluids to help the fiber move through the intestines.

Simple Recipe: Psyllium Digestive Cleansing Drink

Stir 1 teaspoon of psyllium husk into a glass of water or juice. Drink immediately and follow with an additional glass of water to ensure proper hydration and digestive support.

Best Herbs to Use Together

Combine psyllium with licorice root and marshmallow root to soothe and cleanse the digestive tract. Licorice root aids in reducing inflammation in the gut, while marshmallow root provides a mucilaginous coating to ease irritation, making this combination ideal for both cleansing and soothing the digestive system.

HEAVY METAL DETOX

147. Parsley (*Petroselinum crispum*)

Historical Context

Parsley, a common culinary herb, has long been valued for its medicinal properties, particularly in detoxification. Ancient Greeks and Romans used parsley as a garnish and a remedy for various ailments, including its role in purifying the body. In traditional medicine, parsley has been recognized for its ability to support kidney and urinary health, which are critical in detoxification. Modern research has increasingly supported its detoxifying effects, especially in relation to heavy metal cleansing.

Active Compounds and Benefits

Parsley is rich in vitamins A, C, and K, as well as the essential minerals iron and potassium. However, its detoxifying benefits are largely attributed to its high chlorophyll content, which helps to eliminate toxins and heavy metals from the body. Parsley also contains flavonoids and volatile oils, which support the kidneys in filtering out toxins and help the body to excrete heavy metals such as lead, mercury, and cadmium. The herb also supports healthy digestion, which is key in removing toxins from the body efficiently.

Most Potent Method of Ingestion

The most effective way to incorporate parsley for detox purposes is through a daily infusion or tea. A typical daily dosage for parsley as a detoxifying agent ranges from 1–2 teaspoons of dried parsley or 1 tablespoon of fresh parsley in teas or smoothies. For tinctures or extracts, 20–30 drops per day may be used, depending on concentration.

Simple Recipe: Parsley Cleanse

For a cleansing drink, steep 1 tablespoon of fresh parsley in hot water for 5–10 minutes, then strain. Add lemon juice and honey for extra detox benefits and to enhance the flavor. Drink this infusion once or twice daily.

Best Herbs to Use Together

Parsley works synergistically with cilantro to enhance heavy metal detoxification, because cilantro helps to mobilize toxins from tissues, and parsley assists in their elimination via the kidneys. Adding dandelion root to this blend can further support liver detox and enhance the cleansing process.

148. Cilantro (*Coriandrum sativum*)

Historical Context

Cilantro, also known as "coriander" in some parts of the world, has been used for thousands of years across various cultures for both culinary and medicinal purposes. In ancient Egypt, cilantro was even used in embalming practices, and in traditional Indian medicine, it was revered for its digestive and detoxifying properties. Today, cilantro is well known for its ability to help the body detoxify from heavy metals, particularly mercury and lead.

Active Compounds and Benefits

Cilantro contains a range of beneficial compounds, including flavonoids, phenolic acids, and essential oils, which contribute to its detoxifying effects. The herb has been shown to bind to heavy metals like mercury, arsenic, and lead, helping to mobilize and remove them from the body. Cilantro also has antioxidant properties, which aid in neutralizing free radicals, reducing oxidative stress, and supporting overall detoxification. Additionally, cilantro can support digestion and promote liver function, both of which are key to the body's natural detox processes.

Most Potent Method of Ingestion

Cilantro is most effective when consumed fresh, either in salads, juices, or smoothies. It can also be made into a tincture or used in herbal teas, although consuming the fresh herb is thought to offer the most potent effects for heavy metal detoxification. Fresh cilantro can be consumed in abundance, adding a handful of leaves to your daily meals or smoothies. For tinctures, take 1–2 ml of a cilantro tincture 2–3 times daily.

Simple Recipe: Cilantro Detox Smoothie

Blend a handful of fresh cilantro leaves with 1 cup of coconut water, 1 small cucumber, a squeeze of lemon, and a tablespoon of chia seeds. Drink daily for a refreshing detox boost.

Best Herbs to Use Together

Cilantro pairs well with zeolite for a potent heavy-metal detox combination. Zeolite helps trap the metals, while cilantro helps to remove them from the body, making them a powerful duo for detoxification.

SKIN DETOXIFICATION

149. Pine Needles (*from Pinus sylvestris*)

Historical Context

Pine needles have long been used in traditional medicine. They were valued for their purifying and protective properties. Native American and European cultures used pine needles to support the respiratory system and skin health and steam baths to cleanse the skin. Revered for their invigorating scent and healing potential, pine needles have recently regained popularity in skin detoxification rituals.

Active Compounds and Benefits

Pine needles contain high levels of vitamins A and C, along with antioxidants and essential oils that help protect and rejuvenate the skin. Their potent antibacterial and anti-inflammatory properties support a balanced skin microbiome, while their vitamin C content promotes collagen production, leading to healthier, more resilient skin. Pine needle oil is particularly effective in detoxifying the skin from pollutants and irritants, helping to soothe and purify it.

Most Potent Method of Use

Pine needle oil is often used in skin-care applications, typically diluted in carrier oils or added to baths for deep detoxification. A pine needle steam inhalation or facial steam can also open the pores, allowing impurities to release while infusing the skin with pine's beneficial compounds.

Simple Recipe: Pine Needle Facial Steam

Add a handful of fresh pine needles or 3–4 drops of pine essential oil to a bowl of hot water. Lean over the bowl with a towel covering your head to trap the steam. Breathe deeply for 5–10 minutes, letting the steam purify your skin and clear your respiratory system.

Best Herbs to Use Together

Combine pine needles with chamomile or lavender for enhanced calming effects, especially in facial steams or bath soaks, because they work together to soothe and detoxify the skin.

150. Kale (*Brassica oleracea*)

Historical Context

Known for its nutritional benefits, kale has roots dating back to ancient Greece and Rome, where it was prized as a healing food. Its rich nutrient profile has made it a staple in detox diets across cultures. In recent years, kale has gained prominence in the wellness community for its profound ability to nourish and cleanse the skin, both from the inside and out.

Active Compounds and Benefits

Kale is loaded with vitamins A, C, and K, and the antioxidant beta-carotene, which help repair damaged skin cells and protect against oxidative stress. Its high chlorophyll content supports natural detoxification pathways in the liver, promoting clearer skin. Sulfur in kale helps the body produce collagen, strengthening skin and promoting a vibrant complexion.

Most Potent Method of Use

Kale works best as a detoxifying ingredient in both topical and internal forms. It can be juiced for a potent drink to support liver function or blended into face masks for topical application, directly imparting its nutrients to the skin.

Simple Recipe: Kale and Green Clay Face Mask

Blend 2 tablespoons of fresh kale leaves with 1 tablespoon of green clay and a small amount of water until it forms a smooth paste. Apply to the face, leave on for 10–15 minutes, and rinse off with warm water. This mask detoxifies, nourishes, and revitalizes the skin.

Best Herbs to Use Together

Kale pairs well with dandelion and nettle in teas or smoothies, because they work synergistically to cleanse the liver, enhancing skin clarity from the inside out.

LYMPHATIC SYSTEM SUPPORT

151. Poke Root (*Phytolacca americana*)

Historical Context

Poke root has a storied history in North American folk medicine, where it was commonly used by Indigenous peoples for its powerful cleansing effects, particularly in supporting the lymphatic system. Traditionally applied in poultices or tinctures, poke root was a staple remedy for conditions thought to involve "stagnation" within the body, especially within the lymph nodes and tissues.

Active Compounds and Benefits

Poke root contains triterpenoid saponins, alkaloids, and phytolaccatoxin, which are compounds known to stimulate lymphatic flow and immune function. It aids in clearing waste from lymph nodes, helping to reduce swelling and inflammation in the lymphatic tissue. Due to its potency, poke root is often used sparingly to help stimulate detoxification, particularly in cases of sluggish lymph flow or swollen lymph glands.

Most Potent Method of Use

Poke root is most effective in small, controlled doses, typically as a diluted tincture. A professional consultation is often recommended due to its strength, because poke root can be toxic in large amounts. Its use as a topical poultice can also provide localized lymphatic stimulation, particularly in cases of swollen glands.

Simple Recipe: Poke Root Lymphatic Tincture

Mix 5–10 drops of poke root tincture with a glass of water, taking no more than twice per day for short durations. This tincture stimulates lymphatic movement but should be used cautiously.

Best Herbs to Use Together

Poke root combines well with red clover and cleavers for enhanced lymphatic support. These herbs help promote gentle detoxification and support immune resilience.

152. Juniper Berries (*Juniperus communis*)

Historical Context

Revered by ancient Greeks, Romans, and Indigenous North American tribes, juniper berries were traditionally used to purify the body and ward off infections. Juniper's distinctive, aromatic berries were also considered sacred, burned as incense to cleanse spaces and used in infusions to support lymphatic and kidney health.

Active Compounds and Benefits

Juniper berries contain powerful essential oils, flavonoids, and terpenes, especially terpinen-4-ol, which is known to enhance lymphatic drainage and improve kidney function. They possess diuretic properties, helping the body to flush out excess fluids and toxins, which can reduce congestion in the lymphatic system and relieve puffiness.

Most Potent Method of Use

Juniper berries can be used in an infusion or steam inhalation. Both methods allow the essential oils to penetrate tissues, supporting lymphatic circulation. Topical application in the form of diluted juniper oil may also stimulate local lymph flow and alleviate joint stiffness.

Simple Recipe: Juniper Berry Detox Tea

Steep 1 teaspoon of dried juniper berries in a cup of boiling water for 10 minutes. Drink once a day to promote gentle detoxification and lymphatic drainage.

Best Herbs to Use Together

Pair juniper berries with dandelion and nettle, which support kidney and lymphatic function, enhancing the body's natural detoxification pathways.

BLOOD PURIFICATION

153. Red Raspberry Leaf (*Rubus idaeus*)

Historical Context

A beloved plant in European and Native American traditions, red raspberry leaf has been used for centuries as a gentle yet powerful blood purifier and women's health tonic. Known for its nutritive and cleansing properties, it has long been valued for its ability to support the blood, liver, and reproductive system, often brewed as a tea to promote vitality and well-being.

Active Compounds and Benefits

Rich in vitamins A, C, and E, as well as tannins and flavonoids, red raspberry leaf helps purify the blood by promoting liver health and supporting the body's natural detoxification processes. Its astringent tannins bind to toxins, while its high mineral content replenishes the body. The leaf also contains fragarine, which can help tone and strengthen the uterine and vascular systems, supporting circulation.

Most Potent Method of Use

Red raspberry leaf tea is one of the most effective ways to extract its purifying properties. The infusion gently releases nutrients, making it ideal for daily support without overwhelming the system. Capsules are also available for those who prefer not to drink herbal teas.

Simple Recipe: Red Raspberry Leaf Purifying Tea

Add 1–2 teaspoons of dried red raspberry leaf to a cup of boiling water and steep for 10–15 minutes. Consume once or twice daily to support blood and liver health.

Best Herbs to Use Together

Combine with nettle and dandelion for enhanced blood purification and nutrient support, creating a synergistic blend that benefits both the liver and kidneys.

154. Pomegranate (*Punica granatum*)

Historical Context

Pomegranate's reputation as a "fruit of life" stretches back to ancient Egypt and the Middle East, where it was revered for its healing and cleansing properties. Rich in symbolism, this fruit was often used in ceremonies and tonics aimed at renewing vitality and purifying the blood. In Ayurvedic and Unani traditions, pomegranate has been cherished for its rejuvenating effects.

Active Compounds and Benefits

Pomegranate is rich in punicalagins, anthocyanins, and ellagic acid, which are potent antioxidants that reduce oxidative stress and support cardiovascular health. These compounds help to clear toxins from the blood, reduce inflammation, and promote overall cellular health. Pomegranate is also known to improve blood lipid profiles, making it valuable for maintaining balanced cholesterol and supporting circulation.

Most Potent Method of Use

Fresh pomegranate juice offers the most potent blood-purifying effects. Consuming the fruit in its whole form also provides fiber, which aids digestion and enhances the body's detoxification processes. Supplements and extracts can also be used for a concentrated intake of its active compounds.

Simple Recipe: Pomegranate Blood Cleanser Juice

Juice one fresh pomegranate and mix with a splash of water or other juice for taste. Drink half a cup daily to promote healthy blood and cardiovascular support.

Best Herbs to Use Together

Pomegranate pairs well with ginger and turmeric, herbs that further support blood purification and circulation, creating a robust blend for anti-inflammatory and antioxidant benefits.

CELLULAR DETOX

155. Nettle Leaf (*Urtica dioica*)

Historical Context

Nettle has a rich history across Europe, Asia, and North America as both a food and a medicinal herb. Used for centuries in traditional medicine, nettle was prized for its blood-cleansing properties and ability to revitalize the body. It has been a staple in detox regimens due to its ability to support organ function, nourish tissues, and promote overall health.

Active Compounds and Benefits

Packed with vitamins A, C, and K, and minerals such as iron, calcium, and magnesium, nettle leaf fortifies cellular health by providing essential nutrients that help the body naturally detoxify. It contains chlorophyll, which aids in eliminating toxins and supports cellular regeneration. Nettle's anti-inflammatory compounds, like quercetin, also reduce oxidative stress, supporting cell health and promoting energy.

Most Potent Method of Use

A daily nettle infusion offers sustained cellular nourishment and detoxification. Capsules and tinctures are also effective but lack the hydration benefits that an infusion provides. When taken regularly, nettle tea is a gentle yet potent cellular cleanser.

Simple Recipe: Nettle Cellular Detox Tea

Place 1–2 tablespoons of dried nettle leaves in a jar, fill with boiling water, and steep for 4–8 hours. Strain and drink 1–2 cups daily to support cellular detox and overall vitality.

Best Herbs to Use Together

Nettle pairs well with dandelion and burdock for comprehensive detoxification, because these herbs provide additional support for the liver and kidneys, enhancing the body's ability to cleanse at a cellular level.

156. Beetroot (*Beta vulgaris*)

Historical Context

Revered by ancient civilizations from the Mediterranean to Mesopotamia, beetroot has long been recognized for its blood-purifying and restorative qualities. Romans and Greeks valued it not only as food but also as medicine to support liver health and boost energy. Beetroot remains popular in modern detox diets for its liver and cellular benefits.

Active Compounds and Benefits

Beetroot is rich in betalains, pigments with powerful antioxidant and anti-inflammatory properties that support cellular detoxification. It also contains nitrates, which enhance blood flow, and betaine, which assists liver function, promoting toxin breakdown and elimination. Additionally, the high iron content in beetroot supports oxygen delivery to cells, promoting cellular vitality.

Most Potent Method of Use

Beetroot juice is one of the most effective ways to harness its detoxifying power, allowing for rapid absorption of its active compounds. It can also be consumed in powder form or added to smoothies for a nutrient boost.

Simple Recipe: Beetroot Cellular Cleanse Juice

Blend or juice one small beetroot with half an apple and a splash of lemon juice. Drink daily to support liver function and cellular health.

Best Herbs to Use Together

Beetroot pairs well with milk thistle and turmeric, herbs known to support liver health and reduce inflammation, making them excellent companions in a cellular detox regimen.

HERBAL REMEDY VIDEO TUTORIALS BELOW!

Hi there! It's Ava again, are you enjoying the recipes so far?..

Experience Herbalism Like Never Before:

Reading about herbal treatments is insightful, but seeing them crafted and applied is another experience entirely. That's why I've developed an exclusive video playlist that delves into specific ailments and the herbal remedies that can alleviate them. Over the years, I've documented effective, easy-to-follow demonstrations that will enhance your skills and confidence in using herbal medicine.

bit.ly/homeapothecary2025

Here is a small portion of what is in the playlist:

- **Joint and Muscle Relief:** Discover herbs that reduce inflammation and soothe aches.
- **Immune Boosting:** Learn to make blends that fortify your immune system.
- **Stress and Anxiety Reduction:** See how certain herbs can calm your mind and improve sleep.
- **Digestive Health:** Follow recipes that improve digestion and soothe gastrointestinal issues.
- **Heart Health:** Understand the benefits of herbs that support cardiovascular function.
- **Additional Remedies:** Dive into treatments for skin conditions, allergies, and more.

Why Watch the Videos?

- **Practical Demonstrations:** See the textures, colors, and techniques in real time—perfect for visual learners.
- **Detailed Explanations:** Understand the 'why' behind each method, enhancing your ability to replicate and adapt recipes.
- **Personal Touch:** Feel connected as I share personal tips and stories from many years of experience.

Get Started Now!

Get comfortable, set up your herbal workstation, and start watching today to bring the power of nature right into your home! Scan the QR code or use the link to start watching today.

Happy Healing,

Ava

HERBS FOR DETOXIFICATION

CLEANSING FROM ENVIRONMENTAL TOXINS

157. Wood Sorrel (*Oxalis stricta*)

Historical Context

Wood sorrel has a storied history in North America, Europe, and Asia, where Indigenous tribes and herbalists valued it as a cleansing and revitalizing herb. Known for its tangy, lemon-like flavor, it has been used as a refreshing tonic to alleviate heat and fatigue and promote internal cleansing, particularly beneficial in environments prone to pollution.

Active Compounds and Benefits

Rich in vitamin C, oxalic acid, and flavonoids, wood sorrel aids in detoxifying the body by neutralizing free radicals and supporting liver function. Its antioxidant properties help scavenge pollutants and protect cells from environmental damage. Additionally, its mild diuretic effect encourages the elimination of toxins through the kidneys, making it a gentle yet effective detox herb.

Most Potent Method of Use

Fresh wood sorrel leaves can be consumed in salads, added to smoothies, or used as a garnish in soups to maximize nutrient intake. Alternatively, a mild infusion offers a more concentrated dose of its detoxifying compounds and is a simple way to incorporate it into daily detox routines.

Simple Recipe: Wood Sorrel Detox Infusion

Place a handful of fresh wood sorrel leaves in a mug, pour boiling water over them, and steep for 10 minutes. Strain and sip to enjoy its mild detoxifying properties.

Best Herbs to Use Together

Wood sorrel combines well with dandelion and chickweed, both of which support liver and kidney function, creating a comprehensive detox blend to help combat environmental toxins.

158. Green Tea (*Camellia sinensis*)

Historical Context

Originating from ancient China, green tea has been celebrated for millennia as a health tonic, energizing drink, and detoxifying agent. Revered by Japanese monks, it was considered a spiritual aid, with its subtle cleansing effect bringing mental clarity and supporting body balance. Today, green tea is esteemed for its antioxidant power in protecting against environmental pollutants.

Active Compounds and Benefits

Green tea is rich in catechins, particularly EGCG (epigallocatechin gallate), a potent antioxidant that neutralizes free radicals and enhances detoxification. It boosts liver enzyme activity, supporting the body's natural detox processes, while also aiding in DNA repair and cellular health. The presence of chlorophyll in green tea further aids in removing heavy metals and toxins from the bloodstream.

Most Potent Method of Use

Consumed as a freshly brewed tea, green tea delivers its antioxidants in their most potent form. Capsules or powdered matcha are alternative methods, offering a more concentrated dose of catechins for those requiring an intense detox.

Simple Recipe: Green Tea Antioxidant Elixir

Steep one teaspoon of high-quality green tea leaves or a matcha powder in hot water (not boiling) for 2–3 minutes. Strain and enjoy 1–2 cups daily for optimal detoxification benefits.

Best Herbs to Use Together

Green tea pairs well with milk thistle and holy basil, two herbs that further support the liver and amplify antioxidant defense, making it an excellent choice for those facing environmental toxins.

DETOXIFICATION FOR WEIGHT LOSS

159. Bitter Melon (*Momordica charantia*)

Historical Context

Bitter melon, a tropical vine native to Africa and Asia, has been used for centuries in traditional medicine systems like Ayurveda and traditional Chinese medicine for its potent detoxifying and weight-loss properties. In many cultures, it is revered as a "miracle fruit" for its ability to cleanse the body, regulate blood sugar, and support metabolic health, making it a staple in herbal weight management regimens.

Active Compounds and Benefits

Bitter melon contains momordicin, charantin, and polypeptide-p, which are compounds known for their hypoglycemic and metabolic-boosting effects. These compounds help regulate blood sugar levels by enhancing insulin sensitivity and promoting glucose uptake by cells, which supports weight loss by reducing fat storage. Additionally, bitter melon has detoxifying properties that aid liver function, help eliminate toxins, and promote overall metabolic efficiency, contributing to healthy weight management.

Most Potent Method of Ingestion

Bitter melon is most effective when consumed as a juice or in capsule form. The juice provides a concentrated dose of its active compounds, while capsules offer a convenient way to incorporate it into daily routines. Cooking bitter melon in meals is also a common way to consume it, although this may reduce some of its potency. For juice, consume 30–60 ml daily, preferably on an empty stomach. For capsules, follow the manufacturer's instructions, typically 500 mg taken twice daily. Regular intake is recommended for optimal weight-loss support.

Simple Recipe: Bitter Melon Detox Smoothie

Blend 1 cup of bitter melon juice with 1 banana, a handful of spinach, and half a teaspoon of ginger powder. Drink daily to support detoxification and weight loss.

Best Herbs to Use Together

Combine bitter melon with green tea, which enhances its metabolic and detoxifying effects, creating a synergistic blend for effective weight loss and body cleansing.

160. Yerba Mate (*Ilex paraguariensis*)

Historical Context

Yerba mate is a traditional South American drink, particularly popular in countries such as Argentina, Brazil and Paraguay. Used for centuries by the Guaraní people, yerba mate was and still is consumed for its energizing and detoxifying properties. Its role as a social and ceremonial beverage has cemented its place in cultures as a health-promoting herb, especially for its benefits in weight loss and metabolic health.

Active Compounds and Benefits

Yerba mate is rich in caffeine, theobromine, and polyphenols, which provide both stimulant and antioxidant effects. The caffeine content boosts metabolism and increases fat oxidation, supporting weight loss by enhancing energy expenditure. The polyphenols in yerba mate help detoxify the body by neutralizing free radicals and promoting liver function. Additionally, yerba mate improves digestion and reduces appetite, aiding in calorie control and consistent weight management.

Most Potent Method of Ingestion

The most traditional and potent method of consuming yerba mate is as a brewed tea, steeped in hot water and sipped throughout the day. It can also be taken in extract or capsule form for a more concentrated dose, or added to smoothies for added energy and detox benefits. Drink 1–2 cups of yerba mate tea daily, or take 500 mg of yerba mate extract up to three times daily. When using capsules, follow the manufacturer's recommended dosage.

Simple Recipe: Yerba Mate Energy Boost Tea

Add 1 tablespoon of dried yerba mate leaves to a mate gourd or teapot. Pour hot (not boiling) water over the leaves and steep for 5–10 minutes. Sip slowly throughout the day to support energy levels and weight loss.

Best Herbs to Use Together

Yerba mate pairs well with *Garcinia cambogia*, which helps suppress appetite and inhibit fat production, enhancing the weight-loss and detoxification effects of yerba mate for a comprehensive weight management strategy.

HERBS FOR HORMONAL IMBALANCES

SUPPORTING MENOPAUSE

161. Red Sage (*Salvia miltiorrhiza*)

Historical Context

Known in traditional Chinese medicine as *Danshen*, red sage has been used for thousands of years to support women's health, especially during menopause. Celebrated for its cooling and balancing effects, red sage has been historically utilized to ease symptoms such as hot flashes, night sweats, and mood swings, helping women through hormonal transitions with greater comfort.

Active Compounds and Benefits

Red sage is rich in tanshinones, salvianolic acids, and flavonoids, which are powerful antioxidants that support cardiovascular health and reduce inflammation. These compounds are especially beneficial for menopausal women, because they protect against oxidative stress and balance estrogen levels, which can fluctuate during this stage. The herb also promotes circulation, addressing symptoms like joint pain and heart palpitations commonly experienced during menopause.

Most Potent Method of Ingestion

Red sage is most effective as a tea or tincture, allowing its calming and circulatory benefits to be absorbed efficiently. When taken daily, it provides gentle, ongoing support for managing menopausal symptoms. For tinctures, take 1–2 ml up to three times daily. For tea, consume 1–2 times a day.

Simple Recipe: Red Sage Menopause Tea

Steep 1–2 teaspoons of dried red sage leaves in 8 ounces of hot water for 10–15 minutes. Add honey or lemon to taste, if desired. Drink twice daily to support hormonal balance and relieve symptoms.

Best Herbs to Use Together

Red sage combines well with black cohosh and Dong Quai to provide comprehensive support for menopausal symptoms, offering relief from hot flashes, mood swings, and other discomforts associated with hormonal changes.

162. Alfalfa (*Medicago sativa*)

Historical Context

Alfalfa has long been used in herbal traditions for its nourishing, hormone-supporting properties. Known as "the father of all foods," this nutrient-rich plant has roots in ancient Persia, where it was prized for both human health and agricultural purposes. Alfalfa's mineral-rich profile made it an essential remedy for vitality and strength, supporting women through all stages of life, especially during menopause.

Active Compounds and Benefits

Alfalfa is high in phytoestrogens, saponins, and essential vitamins such as vitamin K, calcium, and magnesium. The phytoestrogens mimic natural estrogen in the body, helping to balance hormones during menopause. Its mineral content supports bone health, a crucial benefit because women face higher risks of osteoporosis post-menopause. Alfalfa's saponins also aid in cholesterol regulation, making it heart-friendly as well.

Most Potent Method of Ingestion

Alfalfa is most effective as a fresh juice, capsule, or infusion. Consuming it regularly helps maintain hormonal balance, supports bone health, and reduces menopausal discomforts. Take 1–2 grams of alfalfa capsules up to twice daily. Alternatively, drink one cup of alfalfa tea or juice per day to experience its benefits.

Simple Recipe: Alfalfa Infusion

Add 1–2 teaspoons of dried alfalfa leaves to a cup of boiling water and steep for 10 minutes. Strain and drink once daily to support hormone balance and bone strength during menopause.

Best Herbs to Use Together

Alfalfa pairs well with red clover and sage to provide a blend of phytoestrogens and minerals that strengthen the body, balance hormones, and reduce menopausal symptoms effectively.

MANAGING PREMENSTRUAL SYMPTOMS

163. Nigella Seeds (*from Nigella sativa*)

Historical Context

Revered as "the seed of blessing," nigella seeds (also known as "black seed") have been used in Middle Eastern, African, and Asian healing traditions for thousands of years. Nigella seeds were renowned for easing menstrual irregularities, and has been traditionally used to alleviate PMS symptoms, bringing calm and balance to women's monthly cycles.

Active Compounds and Benefits

Nigella seeds are rich in thymoquinone, nigellone, and other essential oils that provide potent anti-inflammatory and antioxidant effects. These compounds work together to reduce cramps, bloating, and mood swings associated with premenstrual symptoms (PMS). Nigella seeds also help regulate blood sugar and hormone levels, which can reduce cravings and stabilize mood during PMS.

Most Potent Method of Ingestion

Nigella seed oil, taken in capsule form or directly by the teaspoon, is one of the most effective ways to experience its PMS-relieving benefits. Alternatively, the seeds can be infused in honey or added to smoothies for easy ingestion. For nigella seed oil, take 1 teaspoon daily or follow dosage instructions on capsule supplements. Start taking a week before menstruation to relieve PMS symptoms.

Simple Recipe: Nigella Seed Honey Infusion

Mix 1 teaspoon of nigella seed powder or a few drops of nigella seed oil with 1 tablespoon of honey. Take once daily, starting 1 week before your period, to reduce PMS symptoms.

Best Herbs to Use Together

Nigella seeds pair well with ginger and fennel, both known for reducing menstrual pain and discomfort. Together, they create a supportive blend for managing PMS symptoms naturally.

164. Blue Cohosh (*Caulophyllum thalictroides*)

Historical Context

A traditional Native American remedy, blue cohosh was historically used to support women's health, especially for managing menstrual irregularities and easing painful cycles. Known as "papoose root" for its role in supporting reproductive health, blue cohosh remains valued for its ability to soothe the symptoms of PMS and aid in hormonal balance.

Active Compounds and Benefits

Blue cohosh contains saponins, alkaloids, and glycosides, including caulosaponin and magnoflorine, which have anti-inflammatory and muscle-relaxing effects. These compounds work effectively to alleviate menstrual cramps and reduce inflammation, helping to relieve PMS symptoms like mood swings, bloating, and breast tenderness.

Most Potent Method of Ingestion

Blue cohosh is most effective as a tincture or decoction, providing concentrated relief from PMS symptoms. Its muscle-relaxing properties are quickly absorbed when taken as a tincture, soothing cramps and tension. Take 10–15 drops of blue cohosh tincture diluted in water up to twice daily. Use sparingly, because high doses can be strong.

Simple Recipe: Blue Cohosh Decoction

Simmer 1 teaspoon of dried blue cohosh root in 1 cup of water for 10–15 minutes. Strain and sip up to twice a day to relieve PMS-related cramps and tension.

Best Herbs to Use Together

Blue cohosh combines well with cramp bark and black cohosh, creating a powerful blend for managing PMS and menstrual pain, because each herb offers unique benefits that support comfort and balance.

BALANCING ESTROGEN LEVELS

165. Kudzu Root (*Pueraria montana*)

Historical Context

Kudzu, a vine native to Asia, has been used for centuries in Chinese medicine for its wide-ranging health benefits. It was known as "the vine that ate the South" due to its rapid growth in the United States, and was cherished for its role in balancing hormones, especially estrogen, and supporting women's health through its natural isoflavones.

Active Compounds and Benefits

Kudzu is rich in phytoestrogens, including daidzein and puerarin, which mimic estrogen in the body, helping to balance hormone levels. These compounds are especially beneficial for women experiencing estrogen fluctuations, because they may help reduce symptoms of estrogen deficiency or imbalance, including mood swings, hot flashes, and irregular cycles.

Most Potent Method of Ingestion

Kudzu root can be taken as a capsule or in powder form, although it also works well in tinctures for fast absorption. Capsules and powders are convenient for consistent dosing, particularly for managing ongoing hormone balance. A typical dose is 500–1,000 mg of kudzu root powder daily or as per the product's directions for capsules.

Simple Recipe: Kudzu Root and Ginger Decoction

Combine 1 teaspoon of powdered kudzu root and half a teaspoon of grated ginger in 1 cup of water. Simmer for 15 minutes, then strain and sip. This decoction supports hormone balance while also aiding digestion.

Best Herbs to Use Together

Kudzu pairs well with black cohosh and Dong Quai for a supportive blend that enhances hormonal balance and eases menopausal or menstrual discomfort.

166. Lady's Mantle (*Alchemilla vulgaris*)

Historical Context

Known as "the woman's herb," Lady's Mantle has been used since the Middle Ages for its ability to support women's reproductive health. Herbalists have long turned to this herb to address menstrual irregularities, reduce heavy bleeding, and support hormonal equilibrium, earning it a place of honor in European folk medicine.

Active Compounds and Benefits

Lady's Mantle contains tannins, salicylic acid, and flavonoids, which help regulate menstrual cycles, reduce menstrual cramping, and balance estrogen levels. Its astringent and anti-inflammatory properties make it effective in addressing hormonal imbalances and supporting reproductive health.

Most Potent Method of Ingestion

Lady's Mantle is best used as an infusion or in a salve for topical application. As an infusion, it works from within to support estrogen balance and menstrual regularity. Topically, it can be used in salves for soothing skin inflammation related to hormonal changes. To make an infusion, steep 1–2 teaspoons of dried Lady's Mantle in hot water for 10 minutes. Drink up to twice daily, especially around menstruation.

Simple Recipe: Lady's Mantle Herbal Bath Soak

Add 1 cup of dried Lady's Mantle to a muslin bag, then steep in a warm bath. This bath soak promotes relaxation and hormone balance, especially soothing for women experiencing PMS or perimenopausal symptoms.

Best Herbs to Use Together

Lady's Mantle pairs well with red clover and raspberry leaf for a powerful blend to support estrogen balance and overall reproductive health. Together, these herbs offer a well-rounded approach to hormonal harmony.

SUPPORTING THYROID FUNCTION

167. Ashitaba (*Angelica keiskei*)

Historical Context

Originating in Japan, Ashitaba has long been treasured in traditional Japanese medicine for its rejuvenating properties. This verdant plant, known as "Tomorrow's Leaf," for its ability to regenerate quickly, is cherished for its support of thyroid function and overall endocrine health, making it a staple in natural remedies for centuries.

Active Compounds and Benefits

Ashitaba is rich in chalcones, unique compounds with antioxidant, anti-inflammatory, and detoxifying properties. Chalcones, along with vitamins B6, B12, and folate, are essential for supporting thyroid health, energy production, and metabolic balance. Additionally, the plant's iron and chlorophyll content aid in increasing vitality and managing fatigue, a common symptom of thyroid dysfunction.

Most Potent Method of Ingestion

Ashitaba is most effective as a powder or capsule to ensure consistent intake. For an energy boost and enhanced thyroid support, it can be added to smoothies or brewed as a warm infusion to gently support the endocrine system. A standard dose of Ashitaba powder is 1–2 teaspoons daily, either mixed into a drink or taken as a capsule.

Simple Recipe: Ashitaba and Ginger Smoothie

Blend 1 teaspoon of Ashitaba powder with 1 cup of coconut water, half a cup of spinach, 1 inch of fresh ginger, and a few ice cubes.

Best Herbs to Use Together

Ashitaba pairs well with Schisandra berry and holy basil to support energy levels, reduce stress, and enhance overall endocrine function, making it a holistic choice for thyroid health.

168. Bladderwrack (*Fucus vesiculosus*)

Historical Context

Bladderwrack, a type of seaweed, has been used in European folk medicine for hundreds of years, especially for supporting thyroid function. Known for its iodine content, bladderwrack has been a mainstay in natural medicine for boosting metabolism and addressing iodine deficiencies, essential for thyroid health.

Active Compounds and Benefits

Bladderwrack contains high levels of iodine, a mineral crucial for producing thyroid hormones. It also provides other minerals like magnesium, calcium, and potassium, which support the thyroid and improve overall metabolic health. The plant's natural alginates help to detoxify the body, providing additional support to the thyroid.

Most Potent Method of Ingestion

Bladderwrack is best taken as a tincture or in powdered form. Tinctures allow for precise dosing, while the powdered form can be added to capsules or smoothies. Due to the potent iodine content, caution is recommended with dosage, particularly for those with thyroid sensitivity. Typical usage is 500–1,000 mg of bladderwrack powder daily or 10–20 drops of tincture, but it's best to consult a healthcare provider for specific needs.

Simple Recipe: Bladderwrack and Turmeric Tincture

Combine 1 teaspoon of dried bladderwrack and 1 teaspoon of dried turmeric root in a small jar. Cover with alcohol and let steep for 2 weeks. Strain and use 10–15 drops daily to support thyroid function and reduce inflammation.

Best Herbs to Use Together

Bladderwrack pairs well with ashwagandha and lemon balm for a blend that supports thyroid function, reduces stress, and improves metabolic balance, promoting holistic thyroid health.

ADRENAL SUPPORT

169. Siberian Rhubarb (*Rheum rhaponticum*)

Historical Context

Siberian rhubarb has roots in ancient European and Asian medicine, where it has been valued for its adaptogenic qualities and support for the body's stress response. Known as a powerful ally for menopausal women, this herb has also been used historically for its tonic effects on adrenal health, helping to balance hormones and energy levels.

Active Compounds and Benefits

Siberian rhubarb contains unique phytoestrogens, primarily rhaponticin and desoxyrhaponticin, which interact gently with the endocrine system to modulate the stress hormone, cortisol. These compounds help ease adrenal fatigue, regulate mood swings, and promote a sense of balance in the body. Its antioxidant properties further aid in reducing oxidative stress, which often burdens the adrenals.

Most Potent Method of Ingestion

The most effective form of Siberian rhubarb is as an extract, because this method captures its active compounds at high potency. Alternatively, capsules offer a convenient way to maintain consistent intake for adrenal support. Commonly, 50–100 mg of standardized Siberian rhubarb extract is taken daily. Always consult a healthcare provider, especially for long-term use or for those with hormonal imbalances.

Simple Recipe: Siberian Rhubarb Extract Capsules

Fill capsules with 100 mg of Siberian rhubarb extract for a simple, effective daily dose to support adrenal balance, reduce fatigue, and manage cortisol levels.

Best Herbs to Use Together

Siberian rhubarb pairs well with holy basil and rhodiola, both adaptogens that enhance adrenal function, reduce stress, and restore energy levels.

170. Amla (*Phyllanthus emblica*)

Historical Context

Amla, or Indian gooseberry, has a long history in Ayurvedic medicine for its rejuvenating effects on the body and its particular ability to nourish the adrenals. Known as a "rasayana," or rejuvenator, Amla has been cherished for centuries for its capacity to support vitality, resilience, and hormonal balance.

Active Compounds and Benefits

Amla is exceptionally high in vitamin C, a critical nutrient for adrenal health because the adrenal glands use it to produce cortisol and other hormones. It also contains antioxidants such as flavonoids and tannins, which protect the adrenal glands from oxidative stress. Amla's adaptogenic properties make it ideal for managing fatigue, supporting energy levels, and promoting a stable mood.

Most Potent Method of Ingestion

Amla is best consumed as a powder or capsule. The powder can be added to smoothies, teas, or taken in capsule form for ease. In Ayurveda, it's also commonly consumed as a jam-like paste called "churna," offering a convenient, concentrated source of Amla. A typical daily dose is 1–2 grams of Amla powder or one tablespoon of Amla churna. It's safe for regular consumption as an adaptogen.

Simple Recipe: Amla Churna Paste

Mix 1 tablespoon of Amla powder with a teaspoon of honey and a splash of warm water. Take this paste daily to support adrenal resilience, enhance immunity, and reduce stress.

Best Herbs to Use Together

Amla pairs well with ashwagandha and licorice root, which also support adrenal health, bolster energy, and help regulate the body's response to stress.

MANAGING POLYCYSTIC OVARY SYNDROME

171. White Peony (*Paeonia lactiflora*)

Historical Context

White peony has been cherished in traditional Chinese medicine for over 1,200 years, often regarded as a tonic herb for women's health. Known for its ability to harmonize the reproductive system, it has been used to address symptoms of hormonal imbalance, including those associated with Polycystic Ovary Syndrome (PCOS).

Active Compounds and Benefits

White peony contains the unique compound paeoniflorin, which helps modulate hormones and support balanced estrogen levels. This herb works to reduce androgen levels, alleviating symptoms of PCOS such as irregular menstruation, acne, and hair loss. Paeoniflorin also has anti-inflammatory and antispasmodic properties, which help relieve menstrual pain and stabilize mood.

Most Potent Method of Ingestion

White peony is highly effective as a tincture or decoction, because these methods best extract its beneficial compounds. In traditional use, decoctions are commonly made with roots to retain their potent effects. Standard dosages for white peony tinctures are around 30–50 drops, taken two to three times daily. Consult with a healthcare professional, especially when used for chronic conditions.

Simple Recipe: White Peony and Ginger Decoction

Simmer 1 tablespoon of dried white peony root and a few slices of fresh ginger in 2 cups of water for 15–20 minutes. Strain and drink twice daily to support hormone balance, reduce inflammation, and manage symptoms of PCOS.

Best Herbs to Use Together

White peony works well with licorice root and Dong Quai for overall reproductive health and hormone balance, because they complement its estrogen-modulating and calming effects.

172. Tribulus (*Tribulus terrestris*)

Historical Context

Tribulus, also known as "puncture vine," has a long-standing place in Ayurvedic and traditional Chinese medicine for supporting fertility, reproductive health, and energy levels. Historically, it has been used as a restorative herb, helping to balance hormones and improve overall vitality.

Active Compounds and Benefits

Tribulus is rich in steroidal saponins, particularly protodioscin, which support hormone balance by modulating the release of luteinizing hormone (LH). For women with PCOS, this can help reduce androgen levels, regulate menstrual cycles, and improve ovulation. Its anti-inflammatory properties further aid in managing symptoms like acne and abdominal discomfort.

Most Potent Method of Ingestion

Tribulus is best taken as a capsule or powder, although a tincture can also be effective. Capsules and powders offer a convenient way to ensure consistent dosing, which is especially important for managing chronic conditions. A typical dose is 500–1,000 mg of Tribulus extract per day. For best results, consult a healthcare provider to tailor dosage based on individual needs.

Simple Recipe: Tribulus Hormone-Balancing Capsules

Fill empty capsules with 500 mg of Tribulus powder. Take one capsule twice daily to support hormone balance, improve menstrual regularity, and alleviate PCOS symptoms.

Best Herbs to Use Together

Tribulus pairs well with saw palmetto and Shatavari for supporting reproductive health, regulating hormones, and reducing PCOS-related inflammation and androgen levels.

SUPPORTING FERTILITY

173. False Unicorn Root (*Chamaelirium luteum*)

Historical Context

False Unicorn Root, also known as "fairy wand," has a long tradition in Native American and folk medicine as a powerful ally in women's reproductive health. Revered as a sacred herb, it was often used by midwives to enhance fertility and support a healthy pregnancy.

Active Compounds and Benefits

This herb contains steroidal saponins, which may play a role in modulating hormones by stimulating the pituitary gland. False Unicorn Root is known to support ovarian function, balance estrogen, and enhance fertility by preparing the uterine lining for conception. Its calming effect on the nervous system also helps alleviate stress, which can impact fertility.

Most Potent Method of Ingestion

False Unicorn Root is most effective as a tincture, allowing for precise dosing and easy absorption of its potent compounds. Traditional preparations often include a decoction, but the tincture is more commonly used today due to its convenience. A standard dosage is around 1–2 ml of tincture up to three times daily. However, it is essential to consult with a healthcare professional when using False Unicorn Root for fertility, because high doses or prolonged use may not be advisable.

Simple Recipe: False Unicorn Root Fertility Tincture

Add 1–2 ml of False Unicorn Root tincture to a glass of water and drink twice daily. This simple tincture can help support ovarian health, regulate hormones, and enhance fertility.

Best Herbs to Use Together

False Unicorn Root pairs well with red clover and Dong Quai, because these herbs synergistically support reproductive health, balance hormones, and improve uterine tone.

174. Chaste Tree Berry (*Vitex agnus-castus*)

Historical Context

Known as the "women's herb," chaste tree berry has been used for thousands of years, particularly in Ancient Greece and Rome, to balance hormones and support fertility. Monks in the Middle Ages used it to promote celibacy, earning it the name "monk's pepper."

Active Compounds and Benefits

Chaste tree berry is rich in iridoid glycosides, particularly agnuside, which influence the hypothalamic–pituitary–ovarian axis. This helps to balance progesterone and estrogen levels, regulate menstrual cycles, and improve ovulation. Chaste tree berry is especially beneficial for women with luteal phase defects or those experiencing irregular cycles.

Most Potent Method of Ingestion

A tincture or capsule is highly effective, offering steady dosing of active compounds. Chaste tree berry takes several months to reach its full effect, so consistency is key when using this herb for fertility. A common dose is 500–1,000 mg of chaste tree berry extract daily, or 1–2 ml of tincture in the morning, because this aligns with the body's natural hormone rhythms.

Simple Recipe: Chaste Berry Balancing Tincture

Take 1–2 ml of chaste tree berry tincture every morning to help balance progesterone, regulate cycles, and support fertility.

Best Herbs to Use Together

Chaste tree berry pairs well with red raspberry leaf and maca root, because these herbs complement its hormone-balancing properties, providing overall support to reproductive health and fertility.

BALANCING TESTOSTERONE LEVELS

175. Saw Palmetto (*Serenoa repens*)

Historical Context

Native Americans, particularly the Seminole tribe, traditionally used saw palmetto berries to support urinary and reproductive health. The berries of this small palm have been utilized for centuries, valued for their ability to enhance vitality and balance hormones in men, especially in the context of aging

Active Compounds and Benefits

Saw palmetto is rich in fatty acids, phytosterols, and flavonoids, which work together to modulate testosterone levels. It inhibits the enzyme 5-alpha-reductase, which converts testosterone to dihydrotestosterone (DHT). This makes it especially beneficial for supporting prostate health and managing symptoms of benign prostatic hyperplasia (BPH). Saw palmetto also helps alleviate hormonal imbalances that can lead to hair loss, acne, and reproductive health issues.

Most Potent Method of Ingestion

Saw palmetto is often taken as a tincture or in capsule form, allowing for consistent and controlled dosing of its active compounds. Both forms are effective; however, a high-quality tincture provides enhanced absorption of its fat-soluble compounds.

Simple Recipe: Saw Palmetto Testosterone-Balancing Tincture

Take 1–2 ml of saw palmetto tincture twice daily, with meals, to support testosterone balance, reduce DHT production, and promote reproductive health.

Best Herbs to Use Together

Saw palmetto pairs well with nettle root and pumpkin seed, because both of these support prostate health and enhance the hormone-balancing effects, especially in men over 40.

176. Pygeum (*Prunus africana*)

Historical Context

Pygeum bark has been used for centuries in African traditional medicine to support urinary and reproductive health. Indigenous communities relied on it for its anti-inflammatory and hormone-balancing properties, particularly in men with prostate issues.

Active Compounds and Benefits

Pygeum contains phytosterols (such as beta-sitosterol) and pentacyclic triterpenes, which are known to reduce inflammation, inhibit the production of DHT, and promote a balanced testosterone level. Pygeum supports prostate health, alleviates symptoms of BPH, and improves urinary function. Additionally, its anti-inflammatory properties make it beneficial for overall hormonal balance in men.

Most Potent Method of Ingestion

Pygeum is most effective when taken as a capsule or tincture, both of which provide a concentrated dose of its active compounds. A daily dose is generally sufficient to experience its benefits over time.

Simple Recipe: Pygeum Prostate-Supporting Tincture

Take 1–2 ml of Pygeum tincture once or twice daily to support prostate health, balance testosterone, and alleviate symptoms associated with BPH.

Best Herbs to Use Together

Pygeum complements saw palmetto and reishi mushroom, creating a potent blend that supports testosterone balance, reduces inflammation, and enhances urinary health, particularly for those dealing with age-related hormonal changes.

REGULATING MENSTRUAL CYCLES

177. Wild Yam (*Dioscorea villosa*)

Historical Context

Wild yam, native to North America, has a rich history in traditional medicine for women's health. Indigenous tribes and early American herbalists used it to address menstrual discomfort and balance hormones, relying on its natural compounds to ease symptoms of irregular cycles.

Active Compounds and Benefits

Wild yam contains diosgenin, a phytosteroid often considered a precursor to progesterone. While it doesn't directly convert to progesterone in the body, it can help maintain hormonal equilibrium, supporting menstrual regularity and easing premenstrual discomfort. Its anti-inflammatory properties also make it useful for alleviating menstrual cramps.

Most Potent Method of Ingestion

Wild yam is most effective as a tincture or capsule for internal hormonal support. The tincture form provides swift absorption, while capsules offer a convenient way to achieve a consistent dose.

Simple Recipe: Wild Yam Hormone-Balancing Tincture

Take 1–2 ml of wild yam tincture once or twice daily to support hormonal balance, promote menstrual regularity, and ease premenstrual discomfort.

Best Herbs to Use Together

Wild yam pairs well with black cohosh and Dong Quai, because these herbs also support hormone balance and menstrual health, creating a synergistic effect for menstrual regulation.

178. Black Haw (*Viburnum prunifolium*)

Historical Context

Black haw has been cherished for centuries in both Native American and European herbal traditions. Historically, it was used to support women's reproductive health, especially to ease menstrual irregularities and alleviate the pain of menstruation. Early settlers used black haw for its uterine tonic properties, particularly to strengthen the uterine muscles and support overall menstrual health.

Active Compounds and Benefits

Black haw contains iridoid glycosides, flavonoids, and alkaloids, which contribute to its muscle-relaxing and anti-inflammatory properties. It is especially known for its ability to tone the uterine muscles, regulate menstrual flow, and alleviate menstrual cramps. By promoting the proper functioning of the uterus, Black haw supports overall menstrual cycle regulation, reducing symptoms such as pelvic discomfort, irregular bleeding, and cramps.

Most Potent Method of Ingestion

Black haw is most effective as a tincture or decoction. The tincture form provides a concentrated dose of the active compounds, while a decoction allows for deep extraction from the bark and roots, which are typically used in formulations. For the tincture, 1–2 ml per day is typical, taken once or twice daily to provide relief from menstrual discomfort and help regulate the cycle. For a decoction, consume one cup 1–2 times daily.

Simple Recipe: Black Haw Uterine Tonic Decoction

Steep 1–2 teaspoons of dried black haw bark in boiling water for 10–15 minutes, strain, and drink 1–2 cups daily to support menstrual health and ease cramps.

Best Herbs to Use Together

Black haw is highly effective when combined with cramp bark for its complementary action in alleviating menstrual cramps and promoting a healthy, regular cycle. Additionally, red raspberry leaf and Vitex can enhance black haw's ability to balance the menstrual cycle and support uterine health.

SUPPORTING POSTPARTUM HORMONE BALANCE

179. Schisandra Berry (*Schisandra chinensis*)

Historical Context

Schisandra, often referred to as the "five-flavor fruit," has been a cornerstone of traditional Chinese medicine for centuries. Its ability to balance and nourish the body made it highly valued for postpartum recovery. In ancient times, Schisandra was used to support overall vitality and harmonize the body's energies after childbirth, aiding in the restoration of balance in the body and mind.

Active Compounds and Benefits

Schisandra is a powerful adaptogen, rich in lignans, antioxidants, and vitamins. It supports hormone balance by nourishing the liver, which is crucial for hormone detoxification and regulation. Schisandra's adaptogenic properties help the body cope with the stress of postpartum recovery while restoring vitality. It also promotes the production of prolactin, supporting healthy lactation and enhancing the body's natural healing process.

Most Potent Method of Ingestion

Schisandra is typically taken as a tincture, extract, or powder. The tincture provides quick absorption, making it a convenient and effective form for postpartum women who need consistent support. Powdered Schisandra can also be added to smoothies or herbal teas. For tincture, 2–3 drops of Schisandra extract can be taken 2–3 times daily. Alternatively, 1–2 teaspoons of powdered Schisandra can be mixed into water or a smoothie once or twice a day.

Simple Recipe: Schisandra Berry Adaptogenic Tonic

Add 1 teaspoon of Schisandra berry powder to hot water or tea. Let it steep for 5–10 minutes and sip throughout the day to support postpartum hormonal balance and restore energy.

Best Herbs to Use Together

Schisandra works well with ashwagandha and holy basil for postpartum recovery due to their complementary adaptogenic properties. Combined with red clover or red raspberry leaf, Schisandra can provide additional support for hormonal balance and reproductive health during the postpartum period.

180. Goji Berry (*Lycium barbarum*)

Historical Context

Goji berries, known as "wolfberries," have a long history of use in traditional Chinese medicine, particularly for boosting vitality and supporting reproductive health. Used for over 2,000 years, goji has been considered a powerful tonic for restoring youthfulness, nourishing the blood, and balancing the body's energy. During postpartum recovery, goji is particularly prized for its ability to strengthen the body and support hormonal recovery.

Active Compounds and Benefits

Goji berries are rich in vitamins, antioxidants, and amino acids. They contain a unique blend of polysaccharides, which are known to stimulate the immune system, promote energy, and balance hormones. In the postpartum period, goji berries help enhance the body's ability to cope with stress, support hormonal regulation, and replenish essential nutrients lost during childbirth. Their ability to nourish the liver and kidneys further aids in detoxification and hormonal balance.

Most Potent Method of Ingestion

Goji berries are commonly consumed in dried form, tincture, or powder. They can be eaten directly as a snack, added to smoothies, or brewed as a tea. For postpartum women, Goji berry extract or tincture provides a concentrated and effective dose to promote recovery and hormone balance. Goji berries can be consumed as a daily snack (1–2 tablespoons), or 1–2 teaspoons of goji powder can be added to a smoothie or tea. As a tincture, 1–2 ml daily is sufficient.

Simple Recipe: Goji Berry Healing Tea

Steep 1 tablespoon of dried goji berries in hot water for 5–10 minutes. Add honey or lemon for flavor. Drink once or twice a day to support hormonal recovery and overall vitality.

Best Herbs to Use Together

Goji berries synergize well with Schisandra and Dong Quai to restore hormonal balance and energy during postpartum recovery. When combined with red clover and milk thistle, goji can help promote liver detoxification and hormonal health.

HERBS FOR MENTAL CLARITY

ENHANCING MEMORY

181. Malkangni (Celastrus paniculatus)

Historical Context

Malkangni, also known as the "Intellect Tree," has been used in traditional Ayurvedic medicine for centuries to enhance cognitive function. It is particularly valued for its ability to support memory, concentration, and mental clarity. This herb has been a cornerstone of brain tonics in India, known for its potential to improve mental health and sharpen the intellect, especially in those experiencing cognitive decline or mental fatigue.

Active Compounds and Benefits

The active compounds in Malkangni, including alkaloids, flavonoids, and essential fatty acids, are believed to nourish the brain and improve blood circulation to the head. These compounds help boost cognitive function, memory retention, and learning capacity by increasing acetylcholine levels, a neurotransmitter vital for memory and brain health. Additionally, it has antioxidant properties that protect the brain from oxidative damage.

Most Potent Method of Ingestion

Malkangni is most effective in tincture form, which allows for the concentrated benefits of its active compounds. It can also be consumed as a powder, added to smoothies, or in capsule form for easier ingestion. Take 1-2 teaspoons of Malkangni powder or 20–30 drops of tincture once or twice daily. Capsules can be taken according to the manufacturer's recommended dosage, typically 1–2 capsules daily.

Simple Recipe: Mental Clarity Tonic

Mix 1 teaspoon of Malkangni powder with honey and a pinch of black pepper. Consume this blend twice a day to enhance focus and cognitive clarity, especially when engaging in demanding mental tasks.

Best Herbs to Use Together

Malkangni pairs well with ginkgo, which improves memory and mental sharpness. Together, they create a powerful remedy for boosting cognitive function.

182. Periwinkle (*Vinca minor*)

Historical Context

Periwinkle has a long history of use in traditional European and Chinese medicine, where it was used to improve circulation and treat a variety of ailments. It was historically used to improve mental sharpness and alleviate memory loss. The herb continues to be a staple in herbal medicine for supporting brain health and memory retention.

Active Compounds and Benefits

Periwinkle contains several alkaloids, including vinpocetine and vincamine, which improve blood flow to the brain, enhance oxygen and nutrient delivery, and support memory and mental clarity. These compounds also possess neuroprotective effects, shielding the brain from oxidative stress and promoting cognitive health. Periwinkle also helps regulate neurotransmitters involved in memory and learning.

Most Potent Method of Ingestion

The most potent way to take periwinkle is in tincture form, which allows for the best absorption of its active compounds. It can also be consumed as a tea or decoction, or in capsule form for easier consumption. Take 20–30 drops of periwinkle tincture 1–3 times daily, or consume capsules according to the manufacturer's recommended dosage, typically 1–2 capsules per day.

Simple Recipe: Periwinkle Brain-Boosting Tea

Steep 1 teaspoon of dried periwinkle leaves in hot water for 5–10 minutes. Drink up to 2 cups per day to support memory and mental sharpness, especially during times of mental fatigue or focus.

Best Herbs to Use Together

Periwinkle works well with Brahmi, an herb known for its cognitive-enhancing properties. Together, they create a robust remedy for improving mental clarity and memory retention.

REDUCING BRAIN FOG

183. Yerba Buena (*Clinopodium douglasii*)

Historical Context

Yerba buena, often referred to as "good herb" in Spanish, has been used for centuries in Indigenous medicine to alleviate various ailments, including headaches, digestive issues, and mental fatigue. Traditionally used by Native American tribes in the Western United States, yerba buena was valued for its soothing properties, particularly in relieving mental fog and promoting clarity of thought. It has long been recognized as an effective remedy for lifting mental sluggishness and refreshing the mind.

Active Compounds and Benefits

Yerba buena contains essential oils, flavonoids, and menthol, which contribute to its stimulating and calming effects. These compounds help to increase circulation to the brain, promoting mental alertness and clarity. Yerba buena is also known to have mild analgesic and antispasmodic properties, which can relieve the tension and discomfort that often accompanies brain fog. By soothing the nervous system and improving blood flow, it aids in reducing mental fatigue and enhancing cognitive function.

Most Potent Method of Ingestion

Yerba buena is most effective when consumed as an infusion or tincture. A strong herbal tea made from the leaves is particularly beneficial for mental clarity. Tincture form also provides concentrated doses for faster results. For tea, drink up to 3 cups per day. For tincture, take 20–30 drops 1–2 times daily, or follow the manufacturer's dosage for capsule forms.

Simple Recipe: Yerba Buena Clarity Tea

Steep 1–2 teaspoons of dried yerba buena leaves in hot water for 5–10 minutes. Drink this tea throughout the day to support mental clarity and reduce brain fog, especially when you need to focus or when experiencing mental fatigue.

Best Herbs to Use Together

Yerba buena pairs well with peppermint to enhance its cognitive effects. Together, they create a refreshing tea that clears the mind and boosts focus.

184. Passion Fruit (*Passiflora edulis*)

Historical Context

Passion fruit, or maracuja, is native to South America and has been used for centuries by Indigenous cultures to treat anxiety, sleep disorders, and mental fatigue. The fruit and its extracts were revered for their calming properties and ability to soothe the mind, providing mental clarity during times of stress and overwhelm. In addition to its culinary uses, passion fruit has long been considered a valuable medicinal plant for its sedative and brain-supporting qualities.

Active Compounds and Benefits

Passion fruit is rich in alkaloids, flavonoids, and vitamins, including vitamin C and carotenoids, which support overall brain health. The fruit has mild sedative effects due to the presence of harman alkaloids, which help to relax the nervous system and alleviate the stress that often contributes to brain fog. It also supports memory and cognitive function by improving circulation to the brain and reducing oxidative stress.

Most Potent Method of Ingestion

Passion fruit is best consumed as a tincture, extract, or in powdered form, which allows for a concentrated dose of its active compounds. The fruit itself can be consumed fresh or in juice form to provide a mild calming effect, especially when consumed in the evening. For tincture or extract, take 20–30 drops 1–2 times daily. To consume fresh fruit, eat one-half to one whole passion fruit per day. For powdered forms, follow the manufacturer's recommended dosage.

Simple Recipe: Passionfruit Brain-Soothing Drink

Blend 1–2 tablespoons of passion fruit powder with a glass of water or coconut water. Drink this refreshing beverage throughout the day to help clear mental fog and promote relaxation.

Best Herbs to Use Together

Passion fruit pairs well with lemon balm to reduce stress and promote mental clarity. Together, they create a calming, brain-boosting combination.

SUPPORTING FOCUS AND CONCENTRATION

185. Stag's-Horn Clubmoss (*Lycopodium clavatum*)

Historical Context

Stag's-horn clubmoss has a long history of use in both traditional Chinese medicine and Western herbalism. The herb has been used for centuries to support mental function, particularly in enhancing memory and cognitive performance. Its active compound, huperzine A, has made it a popular choice in modern herbal formulations for cognitive enhancement.

Active Compounds and Benefits

The primary active compound in stag's horn clubmoss, huperzine A, helps to inhibit acetylcholinesterase, an enzyme that breaks down acetylcholine. By increasing acetylcholine levels, this herb helps to improve memory, concentration, and mental clarity. It is often used to help with brain fog and cognitive decline.

Most Potent Method of Ingestion

Stag's-horn club moss is most commonly consumed as a tincture or in capsule form. The tincture is highly concentrated and provides quicker absorption, while capsules offer a convenient option for daily use. For tincture, take 1–2 ml, 2–3 times daily. The recommended dosage for capsules is typically 50–200 mcg daily.

Simple Recipe: Stag's-Horn Clubmoss Cognitive Enhancer

Combine 1–2 teaspoons of Stag's-horn clubmoss powder in a smoothie or mix into a cup of warm water. Drink once or twice a day to support focus and mental clarity.

Best Herbs to Use Together

Pair Stag's-horn clubmoss with ginkgo for enhanced cognitive performance, because ginkgo improves circulation to the brain, further supporting mental clarity.

186. Skullcap (*Scutellaria lateriflora*)

Historical Context

Skullcap, also known as "blue skullcap" or "mad dog herb" has been used by Native American and European herbalists for centuries to treat anxiety, stress, and neurological conditions. Known for its calming and relaxing effects, skullcap has also gained popularity for supporting mental focus and concentration, particularly in individuals experiencing mental fatigue or stress.

Active Compounds and Benefits

The primary active compounds in skullcap are flavonoids, particularly baicalin, which possess mild sedative and cognitive-enhancing properties. These compounds help to soothe the nervous system, reduce anxiety, and clear mental fog, making it easier to focus.

Most Potent Method of Ingestion

Skullcap is most commonly consumed as a tea, tincture, or capsule. The tincture offers a fast-acting effect, while tea provides a gentler experience. For tea, use 1–2 teaspoons of dried skullcap per cup of boiling water, steeped for 5–10 minutes. For tincture, take 20–30 drops 2–3 times daily.

Simple Recipe: Blue Skullcap Focus Tea

Combine 1 teaspoon of skullcap with 1 teaspoon of lemon balm in hot water. Steep for 5–10 minutes and strain. Drink 1–2 cups per day to support mental endurance and focus.

Best Herbs to Use Together

Skullcap pairs well with lemon balm, which has calming properties and enhances mental clarity.

SUPPORTING COGNITIVE HEALTH IN AGING

187. Chinese clubmoss (*Huperzia serrata*)

Historical Context

Chinese clubmoss has been used in traditional Chinese medicine for centuries, particularly to support cognitive function and improve memory. In modern times, it has gained recognition for its ability to protect against cognitive decline, especially in ageing individuals. The active compound, huperzine A, has been extensively researched for its role in maintaining mental sharpness.

Active Compounds and Benefits

The primary active compound in Chinese clubmoss is huperzine A, which works as an acetylcholinesterase inhibitor. By preventing the breakdown of acetylcholine, a neurotransmitter involved in memory and learning, this herb helps to improve cognitive function, focus, and memory retention. Chinese clubmoss is especially useful for maintaining cognitive health in aging individuals and may even help slow the progression of neurodegenerative diseases like Alzheimer's.

Most Potent Method of Ingestion

Chinese clubmoss is most effective when taken in supplement form, either as a tincture or capsule. The supplement provides a concentrated dose of huperzine A, ensuring maximum absorption and benefit for cognitive support. For huperzine A supplements, the typical dosage is 50–200 mcg per day, depending on individual needs. It is important to follow the specific dosage instructions provided by the manufacturer or a healthcare professional.

Simple Recipe: Huperzia Cognitive Support Tea

Use a small amount of Chinese clubmoss powder (about a quarter teaspoon) and steep it in hot water for 5 minutes. Drink once or twice a day to support cognitive health and mental clarity.

Best Herbs to Use Together

Chinese clubmoss pairs well with ginkgo, which promotes circulation to the brain and enhances cognitive function. This combination helps improve memory and cognitive performance over time.

188. Maidenhair Fern (*Adiantum capillus-veneris*)

Historical Context

Maidenhair fern has a long history of use in both Western and Eastern herbal traditions, particularly for ability to support cognitive health in older adults. Ancient cultures used this delicate fern to help allevia memory loss and to support brain function. This herb was often prescribed for respiratory health in tradition Chinese medicine, but its cognitive benefits have been recognized for centuries.

Active Compounds and Benefits

Maidenhair fern contains a variety of bioactive compounds, including flavonoids and tannins, which he support brain function by improving circulation to the brain and protecting neurons from damage. The compounds also provide mild sedative effects, helping to reduce anxiety and mental stress, which can oft impair cognitive performance.

Most Potent Method of Ingestion

Maidenhair fern is typically consumed as a tea or tincture. The tea is a mild, soothing way to benefit from t herb's cognitive support properties, while tinctures offer a more concentrated form. For tea, use 1–2 teaspoo of dried maidenhair fern per cup of boiling water, steeped for 5–10 minutes. For tincture, take 20–30 dro 2–3 times daily.

Simple Recipe: Maidenhair Fern Memory-Boosting Tea

Steep 1 teaspoon of dried maidenhair fern in 1 cup of boiling water for 5–10 minutes. Strain and enjoy on or twice daily to help support cognitive health.

Best Herbs to Use Together

Maidenhair fern pairs well with ginkgo to improve circulation to the brain and enhance cognitive functio particularly in aging individuals.

REDUCING MENTAL FATIGUE

189. Chaga Mushroom (*Inonotus obliquus*)

Historical Context

Chaga mushroom, a medicinal fungus that grows on birch trees, has been revered for centuries in Siberian and Eastern European cultures. Known for its powerful antioxidant properties, it was traditionally used as a tonic to boost overall health, improve immunity, and combat fatigue. Chaga's medicinal use has spread to the West, where it is valued for its ability to support the body during periods of stress and mental exhaustion. This remarkable fungus has long been regarded as a sacred remedy, believed to help prolong life and enhance vitality.

Active Compounds and Benefits

Chaga mushroom contains a variety of bioactive compounds, including polysaccharides, betulinic acid, and antioxidants such as melanin. The polysaccharides, particularly beta-glucans, are known to stimulate the immune system and help the body resist stress. Betulinic acid has been studied for its anti-inflammatory properties, supporting the body during physical and mental stress. The high antioxidant content in Chaga helps to fight oxidative stress, which is linked to cognitive decline and fatigue. Regular consumption of Chaga can promote sustained energy levels, making it ideal for reducing mental fatigue.

Most Potent Method of Ingestion

Chaga mushroom is most effective when consumed as a tea, decoction, or tincture. A long steeping process is recommended to extract the beneficial compounds. Chaga is also available in powder form, which can be added to smoothies, coffees, or teas. Drink Chaga mushroom tea once a day. For tinctures, 30–40 drops per day are recommended.

Simple Recipe: Chaga Energy Elixir

Add 1 teaspoon of Chaga mushroom powder to 1 cup of hot water and steep for 15 minutes. Stir in honey and cinnamon for added flavor and health benefits.

Best Herbs to Use Together

Chaga pairs well with Siberian ginseng, which is also an adaptogen known to combat fatigue and stress. This combination supports both mental clarity and physical endurance.

190. Kanna (*Sceletium tortuosum*)

Historical Context

Kanna, a succulent plant native to South Africa, has been used for centuries by Indigenous peoples for its mood-enhancing and stress-relieving properties. Traditionally, Kanna was chewed or smoked to reduce anxiety and uplift the spirit. It is often referred to as a "natural anti-depressant" because of its ability to improve mood and mental well-being. In modern herbalism, Kanna has gained popularity for its ability to combat mental fatigue and cognitive decline associated with stress.

Active Compounds and Benefits

Kanna contains alkaloids, particularly mesembrine, which are known for their mood-lifting and cognitive-enhancing properties. These compounds act as serotonin reuptake inhibitors, promoting a sense of calm and reducing feelings of stress. Kanna's ability to regulate mood helps to prevent cognitive decline and fatigue often linked to chronic stress. By elevating serotonin levels, Kanna can improve mental clarity and reduce the mental fog that accompanies mental fatigue.

Most Potent Method of Ingestion

Kanna is most commonly taken in powder or capsule form. It can also be brewed as a tea or consumed as an extract. The powder can be mixed with water or juice for a quick and easy dose. A typical dose of Kanna powder is 50–100 mg per day. For capsules, 1–2 capsules per day are often recommended, depending on the concentration of the extract.

Simple Recipe: Kanna Mood-Boosting Tea

Steep 1 teaspoon of Kanna powder in 1 cup of hot water for 10–15 minutes. Stir in honey for added sweetness and soothing properties.

Best Herbs to Use Together

Kanna works well with rhodiola, another adaptogen that supports cognitive function and reduces fatigue. Combining Kanna and rhodiola helps restore mental balance and alleviate stress-related fatigue.

SUPPORTING MOOD AND COGNITION

191. Sweet Violet (*Viola odorata*)

Historical Context

Sweet violet has been cherished for centuries for its ability to calm the mind and uplift the spirit. In ancient Greece and Rome, it was used not only as a fragrance in perfumes but also as a medicinal herb to alleviate anxiety, depression, and to promote mental clarity. Sweet violet was included in early European herbal remedies, often recommended for its gentle, calming effect on the nervous system. Its soft, purple flowers have symbolized modesty and affection, yet their medicinal uses extend far beyond simple beauty.

Active Compounds and Benefits

Sweet violet contains several bioactive compounds, including flavonoids and saponins, which contribute to its calming and mood-enhancing properties. These compounds help reduce stress and tension by soothing the central nervous system, promoting relaxation without sedating the body. The flower also contains antioxidant properties that may support brain health, improving cognitive function by alleviating mental fatigue and boosting memory retention. Sweet violet's mild sedative effects are ideal for reducing anxiety and promoting a positive mood, which can lead to clearer thinking and better mental focus.

Most Potent Method of Ingestion

Sweet violet is most effective when consumed as a tea, syrup, or tincture. The flowers are gently infused to release their soothing properties. Tinctures offer a more concentrated form and can be taken in small doses throughout the day to keep anxiety and mental stress in check. For tea, drink once or twice a day. For tincture, take 20–30 drops, 2–3 times a day.

Simple Recipe: Sweet Violet Mood-Soothing Tea

Steep 1–2 teaspoons of dried sweet violet flowers in 1 cup of boiling water for 10–15 minutes. Strain and enjoy once or twice a day to help calm the mind and lift your spirits.

Best Herbs to Use Together

Sweet violet pairs well with lemon balm, a gentle herb known for its ability to reduce anxiety and improve mood. The combination promotes relaxation and mental clarity, offering a balanced approach to supporting cognitive function and emotional well-being.

192. Blue Passionflower (*Passiflora caerulea*)

Historical Context

Blue passionflower (not to be confused with *Passiflora incarnata*) has long been valued for its ability to soothe the mind and support emotional health. Native to the Americas, passionflower was used by Indigenous peoples to treat anxiety, insomnia, and nervous disorders. In the 16th century, European settlers brought the plant back with them, where it became widely used as a natural remedy for promoting calmness and supporting sleep. Its striking blue and white flowers have symbolized peace and tranquility, qualities that reflect the plant's medicinal actions on the nervous system.

Active Compounds and Benefits

Blue passionflower contains several active compounds, including apigenin and harman alkaloids, which are known for their calming and mood-boosting effects. These compounds help regulate the neurotransmitters in the brain, including serotonin and GABA, which are essential for emotional balance and cognitive clarity. Passionflower has mild sedative properties that make it particularly effective in reducing anxiety, promoting relaxation, and supporting better cognitive function by reducing stress-related cognitive decline.

Most Potent Method of Ingestion

Blue passionflower is most potent when consumed as a tea, tincture, or capsule. The tea is soothing and can be taken before bed or during stressful moments to enhance mental clarity and calm the mind. For tea, drink during moments of stress. For tincture, 30–40 drops, 2–3 times daily, can provide effective relief from mental fatigue and stress.

Simple Recipe: Passionflower Relaxation Tea

Steep 1–2 teaspoons of dried blue passionflower in 1 cup of boiling water for 5–10 minutes. Strain and sip the calming tea in the evening or during moments of mental stress for cognitive clarity and relaxation.

Best Herbs to Use Together

Blue passionflower pairs well with valerian root, a calming herb that enhances the sedative effects of passionflower, helping to reduce mental fatigue and improve mood. Together, they provide a synergistic effect that soothes the mind and enhances cognitive function.

ENHANCING LEARNING AND RETENTION

193. Spilanthes (*Spilanthes acmella*)

Historical Context

Spilanthes, also known as the "toothache plant" for its numbing effects on the mouth, has a rich history of use in both South America and Africa. Indigenous cultures in the Amazon have used Spilanthes for centuries to treat a variety of ailments, including dental pain and inflammation. More recently, it has garnered attention in herbal medicine for its cognitive-enhancing properties, particularly for its ability to support learning and memory. In Ayurvedic medicine, Spilanthes is also used to support overall brain health and clarity.

Active Compounds and Benefits

Spilanthes contains several active compounds, including spilanthol, which has been shown to have nootropic effects, improving cognitive flexibility and learning retention. It enhances neuroplasticity, helping the brain adapt to new information more efficiently. Spilanthes is also thought to support circulation, which may increase blood flow to the brain, thereby boosting cognitive function. Additionally, the herb's anti-inflammatory properties may protect brain cells from oxidative stress, which could improve memory and concentration over time.

Most Potent Method of Ingestion

The most effective method of consuming Spilanthes is through a tincture or tea. The tincture offers a concentrated form that can be taken throughout the day, while the tea is a milder option that still offers cognitive-enhancing benefits. For tincture, take 20–30 drops, 2–3 times daily. For tea, drink once or twice daily.

Simple Recipe: Spilanthes Cognitive Boosting Tea

Steep 1–2 teaspoons of dried Spilanthes in 1 cup of boiling water for 10–15 minutes. Strain and enjoy once or twice daily to support memory retention and cognitive flexibility.

Best Herbs to Use Together

Spilanthes pairs well with ginkgo, a well-known herb that supports memory and improves brain circulation. Together, these herbs can help enhance cognitive function, particularly in learning and memory retention.

194. Catuaba (*Erythroxylum catuaba*)

Historical Context

Indigenous peoples in Brazil have used Catuaba for centuries, particularly as an aphrodisiac and for its ability to improve memory and mental clarity. The bark of the Catuaba tree was traditionally brewed into teas and consumed for its stimulating and cognitive-enhancing properties. It was also regarded as a powerful tonic for both physical and mental vitality, with tribes in the Amazon associating the herb with strength and endurance. Catuaba continues to be widely used in Brazilian herbal medicine today for its potent effects on mental health and learning.

Active Compounds and Benefits

Catuaba contains alkaloids and flavonoids, which are thought to help stimulate the nervous system, improve circulation, and boost mental clarity. Its cognitive-enhancing effects are attributed to these compounds' ability to support the brain by improving focus, memory, and learning retention. The herb is also believed to protect the brain from oxidative damage, which may help prevent cognitive decline and enhance long-term memory. Catuaba's gentle stimulant effects can improve alertness without causing jitters, making it an excellent choice for sustained focus and learning.

Most Potent Method of Ingestion

Catuaba is commonly consumed as a tea, tincture, or extract. The tea provides a mild, soothing effect, while the tincture offers a more potent and concentrated dose of its cognitive-enhancing properties. For tea, drink once or twice a day. For tincture, take 20–30 drops, 2–3 times daily.

Simple Recipe: Catuaba Brain-Boosting Tea

Steep 1–2 teaspoons of dried Catuaba bark in 1 cup of boiling water for 10–15 minutes. Strain and enjoy once or twice daily to support memory and learning retention.

Best Herbs to Use Together

Catuaba pairs well with rhodiola, an herb known for its ability to enhance mental endurance and memory. Together, these herbs provide a potent combination to improve cognitive function, making them ideal for those looking to boost learning and retention.

SUPPORTING HEALTHY BRAIN FUNCTION

195. Indian Sarsaparilla (*Hemidesmus indicus*)

Historical Context

Indian sarsaparilla has been used in traditional Ayurvedic medicine for centuries. It is renowned for its detoxifying and cleansing properties, often used to purify the blood and support overall vitality. In Ayurvedic practices, it is considered a valuable herb for supporting brain health, because it is believed to clear accumulated toxins from the system, promoting clearer thinking and mental clarity. Traditionally, it has also been used for skin conditions, but its role in enhancing cognitive function has been recognized in modern herbalism.

Active Compounds and Benefits

Indian sarsaparilla contains saponins, flavonoids, and alkaloids, which contribute to its detoxifying and brain-supportive properties. Saponins are known to support the body's natural detox processes, removing impurities from the bloodstream, which can have a positive effect on overall brain health. The herb's anti-inflammatory properties help protect brain cells from oxidative stress, while the flavonoids enhance circulation, ensuring the brain receives the oxygen and nutrients it needs to function at its best. By cleansing the body and supporting healthy blood flow, Indian Sarsaparilla aids in maintaining cognitive function and mental clarity.

Most Potent Method of Ingestion

Indian sarsaparilla is most effective when consumed as a tea or tincture. The tincture offers a concentrated form for more targeted use, while the tea provides a gentler, more soothing option for daily consumption. For tea, take once or twice a day. For tincture, take 20–30 drops, 2–3 times daily.

Simple Recipe: Indian Sarsaparilla Brain-Clearing Tea

Steep 1–2 teaspoons of dried Indian sarsaparilla root in 1 cup of boiling water for 10–15 minutes. Strain and enjoy once or twice daily to support detoxification and promote brain health.

Best Herbs to Use Together

Indian sarsaparilla pairs well with Gotu Kola, a renowned herb in Ayurvedic medicine for supporting cognitive function. Together, these herbs work synergistically to cleanse and nourish the brain, enhancing both mental clarity and memory.

196. Sweet Clover (*Melilotus officinalis*)

Historical Context

Sweet clover has been utilized for centuries in both Western and Eastern herbal traditions. Historically, it was prized for its ability to improve circulation and ease pain, and it was often used in the form of poultices teas to treat various ailments, including poor circulation and stress-related conditions. In more recent yea sweet clover has gained attention for its role in supporting healthy brain function by promoting optimal blo flow to the brain.

Active Compounds and Benefits

Sweet clover contains coumarins, flavonoids, and glycosides, which are compounds known for the circulatory benefits. The herb's primary active compound, coumarin, acts as a natural blood thinn improving circulation and ensuring that oxygen and nutrients reach the brain more efficiently. By improvi circulation, sweet clover helps to enhance cognitive function, mental clarity, and focus. Its anti-inflammato properties also support overall brain health, protecting it from damage due to oxidative stress.

Most Potent Method of Ingestion

The most common method of using sweet clover is as a tea or tincture. The tea is mild and soothing, while t tincture is a more concentrated option for those seeking stronger effects. For tea, drink one or two cups a da For tincture, take 20–30 drops, 2–3 times daily.

Simple Recipe: Sweet Clover Circulation-Boosting Tea

Steep 1–2 teaspoons of dried sweet clover flowers in 1 cup of boiling water for 5–10 minutes. Strain and dri to support circulation and healthy brain function.

Best Herbs to Use Together

Sweet clover works well with ginkgo, an herb known for improving circulation and supporting brain heal Together, they create a powerful combination that promotes blood flow to the brain, helping to mainta cognitive function and mental clarity.

MANAGING ADHD SYMPTOMS

197. Bala Herb (*Sida cordifolia*)

Historical Context
Bala herb is a traditional Ayurvedic herb used for enhancing energy, clarity, and overall mental function. In Ayurveda, Bala is considered a tonic that supports vitality and cognitive function. The herb was popular in India to treat a variety of health issues, including weakness, fatigue, and mental sluggishness. It is particularly valued for its ability to improve focus and attention, making it an excellent remedy for managing ADHD symptoms.

Active Compounds and Benefits
Bala herb contains alkaloids, flavonoids, and glycosides, which contribute to its stimulating and cognitive-enhancing effects. The herb's active compounds help balance the nervous system, improve blood circulation, and enhance brain function. By stimulating the central nervous system, Bala herb increases mental clarity and focus, making it useful for individuals with ADHD who struggle with attention and concentration. Its adaptogenic properties also help the body adapt to stress, which can be beneficial in managing the emotional fluctuations often seen in ADHD.

Most Potent Method of Ingestion
Bala herb is typically consumed as a tincture or powder. The tincture offers a concentrated dose of its active compounds, while the powder can be added to smoothies, teas, or capsules. For tincture, take 20–30 drops, 2–3 times daily. For powder, use quarter to half a teaspoon in a tea or smoothie.

Simple Recipe: Bala Herb Focus-Enhancing Smoothie
Blend half a teaspoon of Bala herb powder with 1 banana, 1 cup of almond milk, and a handful of spinach. Add honey or stevia to taste and enjoy once or twice daily to support focus and attention.

Best Herbs to Use Together
Bala herb pairs well with Brahmi, an herb known for enhancing cognitive function and memory. Together, they create a balanced formula that improves both attention and mental clarity, ideal for managing ADHD symptoms.

198. Cayenne (*Capsicum annuum*)

Historical Context

Cayenne pepper is a well-known spice with a long history of use in both culinary and medicinal practice. Native to Central and South America, cayenne has been used for centuries to treat digestive issues, improve circulation, and stimulate the senses. In modern herbalism, cayenne is often used as a stimulating herb to support focus and concentration. Its ability to increase blood flow to the brain makes it an excellent choice for managing symptoms of ADHD.

Active Compounds and Benefits

The active compound in cayenne, capsaicin, is known for its ability to improve circulation and stimulate the nervous system. Capsaicin enhances blood flow to the brain, ensuring that the brain receives an adequate supply of oxygen and nutrients, which can help improve focus, mental clarity, and cognitive performance. Cayenne also acts as a mild stimulant, helping to boost energy and reduce the mental fatigue often associated with ADHD. Additionally, its anti-inflammatory properties support overall brain health.

Most Potent Method of Ingestion

Cayenne is most commonly consumed as a tincture, powder, or in capsule form. The tincture provides a potent dose of capsaicin, while the powder can be easily added to food or drinks for a milder effect. For tincture, take 10–15 drops, 2–3 times daily. For powder, use a quarter teaspoon mixed with warm water or tea, or take 1 capsule daily.

Simple Recipe: Cayenne Focus-Boosting Tea

Mix a quarter teaspoon of cayenne powder in a cup of warm water or herbal tea. Add honey or lemon to taste and drink once or twice daily to stimulate focus and concentration.

Best Herbs to Use Together

Cayenne pairs well with ginkgo, because both herbs enhance circulation and support cognitive function. Together, they provide a powerful combination for improving focus and managing ADHD symptoms.

PREVENTING COGNITIVE DECLINE

199. Jiaogulan (*Gynostemma pentaphyllum*)

Historical Context

Known as "the herb of immortality" in traditional Chinese medicine, Jiaogulan has been known for its profound health benefits, especially in enhancing longevity and cognitive resilience. Originally used in Southern China, Jiaogulan was prized for its adaptogenic qualities, believed to help the body resist stress and maintain vitality. It has grown popular for its neuroprotective properties, particularly for its role in supporting cognitive health and preventing decline associated with aging.

Active Compounds and Benefits

Jiaogulan is rich in saponins, specifically gypenosides, which are compounds known for their neuroprotective and antioxidant effects. These active compounds support brain health by reducing oxidative stress, enhancing blood flow, and protecting neurons from damage. Additionally, Jiaogulan helps regulate levels of cortisol and other stress hormones, reducing mental fatigue and helping preserve cognitive function over time.

Most Potent Method of Ingestion

Jiaogulan is most effective as a tea or tincture. Consuming it as a tea allows for slow, sustained absorption of its active compounds, supporting daily cognitive function and resilience. The herb is also effective in tincture form, providing a concentrated dose of neuroprotective benefits. Drink 1–2 cups of Jiaogulan tea daily. For tinctures, take 20–30 drops up to three times daily.

Simple Recipe: Jiaogulan Brain-Boosting Tea

Combine 1 teaspoon of dried Jiaogulan leaves with 1 cup of hot water. Steep for 5–10 minutes. Strain and enjoy once or twice daily for cognitive support and to prevent cognitive decline.

Best Herbs to Use Together

Jiaogulan pairs well with ginkgo and Gotu Kola. Together, these herbs enhance circulation to the brain, reduce oxidative stress, and support long-term cognitive health, particularly in aging individuals.

200. Polygala (*Polygala tenuifolia*)

Historical Context

Polygala, also known as "milkwort," has a long tradition in Chinese herbal medicine. Used for thousands years, polygala has been highly valued for its ability to support cognitive health, enhance memory, and preve mental decline. In traditional Chinese medicine (TCM), it is considered a "tonic" for the brain, used to ca the mind, nourish the nervous system, and improve cognitive function. It is often recommended for old adults to support healthy aging and mental clarity.

Active Compounds and Benefits

Polygala contains several bioactive compounds, including saponins and flavonoids, which contribute to cognitive-enhancing properties. These compounds help stimulate the central nervous system, impro memory retention, and promote mental clarity. Polygala also has adaptogenic properties, reducing the imp of stress on the body and mind. Studies suggest that it may support the regeneration of neurons, th preventing the cognitive decline associated with aging. Its calming effects also help alleviate anxiety a mental fatigue, which can impede cognitive function.

Most Potent Method of Ingestion

Polygala is best consumed in the form of a tincture, capsule, or tea. The tincture offers a concentrated form its active compounds, while the powder can be added to smoothies or teas. For tincture, take 20–30 drops, 3 times daily. For capsules, take 500–1,000 mg daily. For tea, drink once a day.

Simple Recipe: Polygala Cognitive-Boosting Tea

Steep 1 teaspoon of dried polygala root in 1 cup of hot water for 5–10 minutes. Strain and enjoy once or tw daily to support brain health and prevent cognitive decline.

Best Herbs to Use Together

Polygala pairs well with Gotu Kola for a powerful cognitive-enhancing combination. Together, they impro memory, mental clarity, and protect against cognitive decline, particularly in aging individuals.

201. Maritime Pine Bark (*Pinus pinaster*)

Historical Context

Maritime pine bark, derived from the bark of the *Pinus pinaster* tree, has a rich history of use in both traditional European and modern herbal medicine. In particular, the French have long used this powerful extract for its health benefits, particularly for improving circulation and promoting cognitive function. It was first popularized as a natural remedy in the 1980s when researchers discovered its potent antioxidant properties. Today, it is widely recognized for its role in supporting brain health and preventing cognitive decline, especially in aging individuals.

Active Compounds and Benefits

Maritime pine bark contains oligomeric proanthocyanidin complexes (OPCs), powerful antioxidants that help protect the brain from oxidative stress and free radical damage. These compounds are known to improve blood flow to the brain, enhance cognitive function, and prevent the deterioration of neurons. Maritime pine bark has been shown to improve memory, learning, and mental clarity by boosting circulation and protecting brain cells. Its neuroprotective effects help reduce the risk of age-related cognitive decline, including conditions such as Alzheimer's disease and other forms of dementia. Additionally, the bark has anti-inflammatory properties that help reduce brain inflammation, a key contributor to cognitive decline.

Most Potent Method of Ingestion

Maritime pine bark is most effective when taken in the form of an extract or capsule. The extract provides a potent dose of OPCs, while capsules offer a convenient way to incorporate it into daily wellness routines. For the extract, take 30–50 mg daily. For capsules, take 100-–200 mg daily.

Simple Recipe: Maritime Pine Bark Cognitive-Boosting Tonic

Add 1–2 drops of maritime pine bark extract to a glass of water or tea. Drink once daily to support brain health and prevent cognitive decline.

Best Herbs to Use Together

Maritime pine bark pairs well with ginkgo, because both herbs promote circulation to the brain and enhance cognitive function. Together, they provide a powerful remedy for preventing cognitive decline and improving mental clarity, particularly in older adults.

HERBAL REMEDY VIDEO TUTORIALS BELOW!

Hi there! It's Ava, and I'm thrilled you're exploring my home apothecary book. Are you enjoying the recipes and remedies? I hope they're inspiring you as much as they've rejuvenated me.

Experience Herbalism Like Never Before:

I understand that sometimes reading about processes isn't quite the same as seeing them in action. That's why I've put together an exclusive video playlist just for you! Over the past decade, I've captured my herbalism journey in detail, and these videos are packed with hands-on demonstrations to enhance your learning and skills.

Here is a small portion of what is in the playlist:

- **Respiratory Health:** Learn steam inhalation techniques for sinus congestion and respiratory ailments.
- **Pain and Wound Care:** Discover compresses and salves that soothe muscle pain, reduce inflammation, and heal skin irritations.
- **Digestive Issues:** See how tinctures can aid digestion, boost immunity, and enhance mental clarity.
- **Throat Relief:** Create lozenges for effective relief from sore throats and coughs.
- **Skin Health:** Follow recipes for salves that address cuts, burns, and other skin issues.
- **Overall Wellbeing:** Gain insights into remedies for headaches, sleep disorders, and stress management.
- **And So Much More:** Explore additional herbal practices and remedies that extend even further into holistic health.

bit.ly/homeapothecary2025

Get Started Now!

Prepare your herbal workstation, and explore deeper into the world of herbalism. Scan the QR code or use the link on this page to access the videos. Start your hands-on learning today and bring the power of nature into every aspect of your health.

Happy Healing,

Ava

HERBAL GLOSSARY

This section provides a quick reference to the herbs featured in the book, organized by the health conditions they support. Each herb is listed under the relevant category, allowing you to easily find information based on your specific health needs.

HERBS FOR DIGESTIVE ISSUES

Soothing Digestive Tract Inflammation

1. Slippery Elm (Ulmus rubra) 40
2. Licorice Root (Glycyrrhiza glabra) 41

Stimulating Digestion

3. Gentian Root (*Gentiana lutea*) 42
4. Artichoke Leaf (*Cynara scolymus*) 43

Relieving Bloating and Gas

5. Caraway (*Carum carvi*) 44
6. Anise (*Pimpinella anisum*) 45

Nausea and Vomiting Relief

7. Meadowsweet (*Filipendula ulmaria*) 46
8. Catnip (*Nepeta cataria*) 47

Balancing Gut Flora

9. Garlic (*Allium sativum*) 48
10. Berberine (*Berberis vulgaris*) 49

Supporting Liver Function

11. Milk Thistle (*Silybum marianum*) 50
12. Schisandra (*Schisandra chinensis*) 51

Constipation Relief

13. Cascara Sagrada (*Rhamnus purshiana*) 52
14. Flaxseed (*Linum usitatissimum*) 53

Diarrhea Management

15. Blackberry Leaf (*Rubus fruticosus*) 54
16. White Oak Bark (*Quercus alba*) 55

Reducing Acid Reflux

17. Mastic Gum (*Pistacia lentiscus*) 56
18. Papaya Leaf (*Carica papaya*) 57

Appetite Stimulation

19. Wormwood (*Artemisia absinthium*) 58
20. Angelica (*Angelica archangelica*) 59

HERBS FOR RESPIRATORY CONDITIONS

Clearing Mucus and Congestion

21. Mullein (*Verbascum thapsus*) 61
22. Elecampane (*Inula helenium*) 62

Soothing Coughs

23. Marshmallow Root (*Althaea officinalis*) 63
24. Wild Cherry Bark (*Prunus serotina*) 64

Reducing Inflammation in the Airways

25. Turmeric (*Curcuma longa*) 65
26. Boswellia (*Boswellia serrata*) 66

Immune Support for Respiratory Health

27. Astragalus (*Astragalus membranaceus*) 67
28. Reishi Mushroom (*Ganoderma lucidum*) 68

Antimicrobial, Anti-inflammatory, Immune Support

29. Goldenseal (*Hydrastis canadensis*) 69
30. Oregano (*Origanum vulgare*) 70

Opening the Airways

31. Lobelia (*Lobelia inflata*) 71
32. Grindelia (*Grindelia robusta*) 72

Relief from Asthma Symptoms

33. Coleus (*Coleus forskohlii*) 73
34. Butterbur (*Petasites hybridus*) 74

Managing Allergies

35. Quercetin (*from various plants*) 75
36. Nettle (*Urtica dioica*) 76

Promoting Lung Health

37. Cordyceps (*Cordyceps sinensis*) 77
38. Yerba Santa (*Eriodictyon californicum*) 78

Reducing Sinus Pressure

39. Horseradish (*Armoracia rusticana*) 79
40. Bayberry (*Myrica cerifera*) 80

HERBS FOR SKIN CONDITIONS

Wound Healing

41. Comfrey (*Symphytum officinale*) 83
42. Plantain (*Plantago major*) 84

Soothing Eczema and Psoriasis

43. Yellow Dock (*Rumex crispus*) 85
44. Evening Primrose (*Oenothera biennis*) 86

Treating Acne

45. Tea Tree (*Melaleuca alternifolia*) 87
46. Holy Basil (*Ocimum sanctum*) 88

Moisturizing Dry Skin

47. Jojoba (*Simmondsia chinensis*) 89
48. Olive Oil (*Olea europaea*) 90

Relieving Burns and Sunburns

49. Aloe Vera (*Aloe barbadensis*) 91
50. Mallow (*Malva sylvestris*) 92

Reducing Scarring

51. Rosehip Seed Oil (*from Rosa canina*) 93
52. Myrrh (*Commiphora myrrha*) 94

Managing Fungal Infections

53. Pau d'Arco (*Tabebuia impetiginosa*) 95
54. Clove (*Syzygium aromaticum*) 96

Reducing Redness and Swelling

55. Witch Hazel (*Hamamelis virginiana*) 97
56. St. John's Wort (*Hypericum perforatum*) 98

Promoting a Healthy Skin Barrier

57. Cocoa Butter (*from Theobroma cacao seeds*) 99
58. Borage Seed Oil (*from Borago officinalis*) 100

Detoxifying the Skin

59. Celandine (*Chelidonium majus*) 101
60. Burdock Root (*Arctium lappa*) 102

HERBS FOR STRESS AND ANXIETY

Calming the Nervous System

61. Skullcap (*Scutellaria lateriflora*) 104
62. Passionflower (*Passiflora incarnata*) 105

Supporting Sleep

63. Valerian Root (*Valeriana officinalis*) 106
64. California Poppy (*Eschscholzia californica*) 107

Balancing Mood

65. Ashwagandha (*Withania somnifera*) 108
66. Rhodiola (*Rhodiola rosea*) 109

HERBS FOR MENTAL CLARITY

Reducing Physical Symptoms of Anxiety

67. Kava (*Piper methysticum*) 110
68. Lemon Verbena (*Aloysia citrodora*) 111

Supporting Adrenal Health

69. Ginseng (*Panax ginseng*) 112
70. Shatavari (*Asparagus racemosus*) 113

Enhancing Mental Clarity

71. Gotu Kola (*Centella asiatica*) 114
72. Brahmi (*Bacopa monnieri*) 115

Reducing Panic Attacks

73. Blue Vervain (*Verbena hastata*) 116
74. Corydalis (*Corydalis yanhusuo*) 117

Supporting Long-Term Stress Management

75. Bay Leaf (*Laurus nobilis*) 118
76. Velvet Bean (*Mucuna pruriens*) 119

Promoting Emotional Well-Being

77. Damiana (*Turnera diffusa*) 120
78. Linden Flower (*Tilia europaea*) 121

Combating Fatigue

79. Maca (*Lepidium meyenii*) 122
80. Suma (*Pfaffia paniculata*) 123

HERBS FOR PAIN MANAGEMENT

Reducing Inflammation

81. Devil's Claw (*Harpagophytum procumbens*) 126
82. White Willow Bark (*Salix alba*) 127

Relieving Headaches and Migraines

83. Feverfew (*Tanacetum parthenium*) 128
84. Skullcap (*Scutellaria lateriflora*) 129

THE COMPLETE HOME APOTHECARY BOOK

Easing Joint Pain and Arthritis

85. Black Cohosh (*Actaea racemosa*) 130
86. Marjoram (*Origanum majorana*) 131

Alleviating Muscle Aches

87. Helichrysum (*Helichrysum italicum*) 132
88. Moringa (*Moringa oleifera*) 133

Soothing Menstrual Cramps

89. Dong Quai (*Angelica sinensis*) 134
90. Motherwort (*Leonurus cardiaca*) 135

Supporting Nerve Health

91. Lion's Mane Mushroom (*Hericium erinaceus*) 136
92. Oat Straw (*Avena sativa*) 137

Topical Pain Relief

93. Arnica (*Arnica montana*) 138
94. Tamanu Oil (*Calophyllum inophyllum*) 139

Managing Chronic Pain

95. Rehmannia (*Rehmannia glutinosa*) 140
96. Sarsaparilla (*Smilax ornata*) 141

Reducing Pain from Injuries

97. Yarrow (*Achillea millefolium*) 142
98. Blue Lotus (*Nymphaea caerulea*) 143

Natural Alternatives to Painkillers

99. Magnolia Bark (*Magnolia officinalis*) 144
100. Hops (*Humulus lupulus*) 145

HERBS FOR IMMUNE SUPPORT

Boosting Overall Immunity

101. Cayenne (*Capsicum annuum*) 147
102. Siberian Ginseng (*Eleutherococcus senticosus*) 148

Preventing Colds and Flu

103. Hyssop (*Hyssopus officinalis*) 149

104. Sage (*Salvia officinalis*) 150

Supporting Recovery from Illness

105. Fenugreek (*Trigonella foenum-graecum*) 151

106. Andrographis (*Andrographis paniculata*) 152

Antiviral Support

107. Neem (*Azadirachta indica*) 153

108. Elderflower (*from Sambucus nigra*) 154

Strengthening Respiratory Immunity

109. Osha Root (*Ligusticum porteri*) 155

110. Coltsfoot (*Tussilago farfara*) 156

Balancing the Immune Response

111. Red Clover (*Trifolium pratense*) 157

112. Blessed Thistle (*Cnicus benedictus*) 158

Supporting Gut-Associated Lymphoid Tissue (GALT)

113. Fennel (*Foeniculum vulgare*) 159

114. Chicory Root (*Cichorium intybus*) 160

Detoxifying the Body

115. Red Root (*Ceanothus americanus*) 161

116. Oregon Grape Root (*Mahonia aquifolium*) 162

Anti-inflammatory Immunity Boosters

117. Agrimony (*Agrimonia eupatoria*) 163

118. Black Walnut (*Juglans nigra*) 164

Adaptogens for Immune Health

119. Ginkgo (*Ginkgo biloba*) 165

120. Spikenard (*Nardostachys jatamansi*) 166

HERBS FOR CARDIOVASCULAR HEALTH

Lowering Blood Pressure

121. Hawthorn (*Crataegus monogyna*) 168
122. Mistletoe (*Viscum album*) 169

Improving Circulation

123. Mugwort (*Artemisia vulgaris*) 170
124. Self-Heal (*Prunella vulgaris*) 171

Reducing Cholesterol

125. Sea Buckthorn (*Hippophae rhamnoides*) 172
126. Fo-Ti (*Polygonum multiflorum*) 173

Supporting Heart Function

127. Saffron (*Crocus sativus*) 174
128. Red Date (*Ziziphus jujuba*) 175

Managing Heart Palpitations

129. Wood Betony (*Stachys officinalis*) 176
130. Chinese Date (*Ziziphus spinosa*) 177

Reducing Inflammation in Blood Vessels

131. Tansy (*Tanacetum vulgare*) 178
132. Fringe Tree (*Chionanthus virginicus*) 179

Supporting Healthy Blood Vessels

133. Dill (*Anethum graveolens*) 180
134. Cardamom (*Elettaria cardamomum*) 181

Managing Varicose Veins

135. Onion (*Allium cepa*) 182
136. Chickweed (*Stellaria media*) 183

Preventing Blood Clots

137. Cranberry (*Vaccinium macrocarpon*) 184
138. Avocado Oil (*from Persea americana*) 185

Promoting Healthy Blood Sugar Levels

139. Cinnamon (*Cinnamomum verum*) 186
140. Cucumber (*Cucumis sativus*) 187

HERBS FOR DETOXIFICATION

Liver Detoxification

141. Chanca Piedra (*Phyllanthus niruri*) 190
142. Bupleurum (*Bupleurum chinense*) 191

Kidney Support

143. Cleavers (*Galium aparine*) 192
144. Corn Silk (*from Zea mays*) 193

Digestive Cleansing

145. Triphala (*combination of Emblica officinalis, Terminalia chebula, and Terminalia bellirica*) 194
146. Psyllium (*Plantago ovata*) 195

Heavy Metal Detox

147. Parsley (*Petroselinum crispum*) 196
148. Cilantro (*Coriandrum sativum*) 197

Skin Detoxification

149. Pine Needles (*from Pinus sylvestris*) 198
150. Kale (*Brassica oleracea*) 199

Lymphatic System Support

151. Poke Root (*Phytolacca americana*) 200
152. Juniper Berries (*Juniperus communis*) 201

Blood Purification

153. Red Raspberry Leaf (*Rubus idaeus*) 202
154. Pomegranate (*Punica granatum*) 203

Cellular Detox

155. Nettle Leaf (*Urtica dioica*) 204
156. Beetroot (*Beta vulgaris*) 205

Cleansing from Environmental Toxins

157. Wood Sorrel (*Oxalis stricta*) 207
158. Green Tea (*Camellia sinensis*) 208

Detoxification for Weight Loss

159. Bitter Melon (*Momordica charantia*) 209
160. Yerba Mate (*Ilex paraguariensis*) 210

HERBS FOR HORMONAL IMBALANCES

Supporting Menopause

161. Red Sage (*Salvia miltiorrhiza*) 212
162. Alfalfa (*Medicago sativa*) 213

Managing Premenstrual Symptoms

163. Nigella Seeds (*from Nigella sativa*) 214
164. Blue Cohosh (*Caulophyllum thalictroides*) 215

Balancing Estrogen Levels

165. Kudzu Root (*Pueraria montana*) 216
166. Lady's Mantle (*Alchemilla vulgaris*) 217

Supporting Thyroid Function

167. Ashitaba (*Angelica keiskei*) 218
168. Bladderwrack (*Fucus vesiculosus*) 219

Adrenal Support

169. Siberian Rhubarb (*Rheum rhaponticum*) 220
170. Amla (*Phyllanthus emblica*) 221

Managing Polycystic Ovary Syndrome

171. White Peony (*Paeonia lactiflora*) 222
172. Tribulus (*Tribulus terrestris*) 223

Supporting Fertility

173. False Unicorn Root (*Chamaelirium luteum*) 224
174. Chaste Tree Berry (*Vitex agnus-castus*) 225

Balancing Testosterone Levels

175. Saw Palmetto (*Serenoa repens*) 226
176. Pygeum (*Prunus africana*) 227

Regulating Menstrual Cycles

177. Wild Yam (*Dioscorea villosa*) 228
178. Black Haw (*Viburnum prunifolium*) 229

Supporting Postpartum Hormone Balance

179. Schisandra Berry (*Schisandra chinensis*) 230
180. Goji Berry (*Lycium barbarum*) 231

HERBS FOR MENTAL CLARITY

Enhancing memory

181. Malkangni (*Celastrus paniculatus*) 233
182. Periwinkle (*Vinca minor*) 234

Reducing Brain Fog

183. Yerba Buena (*Clinopodium douglasii*) 235
184. Passion Fruit (*Passiflora edulis*) 236

Supporting Focus and Concentration

185. Stag's-Horn Clubmoss (*Lycopodium clavatum*) 237
186. Skullcap (*Scutellaria lateriflora*) 238

Supporting Cognitive Health in Aging

187. Chinese clubmoss (*Huperzia serrata*) 239
188. Maidenhair Fern (*Adiantum capillus-veneris*) 240

Reducing Mental Fatigue

189. Chaga Mushroom (*Inonotus obliquus*) 241
190. Kanna (*Sceletium tortuosum*) 242

Supporting Mood and Cognition

191. Sweet Violet (*Viola odorata*) 243
192. Blue Passionflower (*Passiflora caerulea*) 244

Enhancing Learning and Retention

193. Spilanthes (*Spilanthes acmella*) 245
194. Catuaba (*Erythroxylum catuaba*) 246

Supporting Healthy Brain Function

195. Indian Sarsaparilla (*Hemidesmus indicus*) 247
196. Sweet Clover (*Melilotus officinalis*) 248

Managing ADHD Symptoms

197. Bala Herb (*Sida cordifolia*) 249
198. Cayenne (*Capsicum annuum*) 250

Preventing Cognitive Decline

199. Jiaogulan (*Gynostemma pentaphyllum*) 251
200. Polygala (*Polygala tenuifolia*) 252
201. Maritime Pine Bark (*Pinus pinaster*) 253

Made in the USA
Coppell, TX
07 April 2025

47953308R00149